Workbook for

Health Careers Today

Seventh Edition

Judith Gerdin, BSN, MS
Phoenix, Arizona

ELSEVIER

Elsevier
3251 Riverport Lane
St. Louis, Missouri 63043

Workbook for Health Careers Today, SEVENTH EDITION   ISBN: 978-0-323-76462-9

Notices

Knowledge and best practice in this field are constantly changing. As new research and experience broaden our understanding, changes in research methods, professional practices, or medical treatment may become necessary.

Practitioners and researchers must always rely on their own experience and knowledge in evaluating and using any information, methods, compounds, or experiments described herein. In using such information or methods, they should be mindful of their own safety and the safety of others, including parties for whom they have a professional responsibility.

Director, Content Development: Ellen Wurm-Cutter
Senior Content Strategist: Linda Woodard
Senior Content Development Specialist: Kathleen Nahm
Publishing Services Manager: Deepthi Unni
Project Manager: Janish Aswin Paul
Cover Designer: Muthukumaran Thangaraj

Printed in the United States of America

Last digit is the print number: 9   8   7   6   5   4   3   2

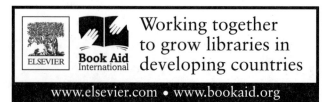

Preface to the Student

This workbook was designed for use with the textbook *Health Careers Today, 7ᵗʰ Edition*. It provides exercises and activities that reinforce the information presented in the textbook and allows you multiple opportunities to demonstrate that content and skill. In this edition, we have revised the text to offer an understanding of the healthcare industry, the different healthcare professions, the skills required to work in health care, and an overview of the work performed by the many professionals who provide patient care and support the healthcare industry.

The chapters of the workbook are divided into the following sections:

- **Knowledge Check** – To reinforce your understanding of the content presented in the chapter. This includes multiple choice and True/False questions.

- **Careers** – To encourage a detailed understanding of the work of healthcare professionals, and the education, skills, and qualities it takes to pursue a career in the field.

- **Content Instruction** – Assessments of the content relating to the knowledge base of the healthcare professionals discussed in the chapter.

- **Performance Instruction** – "Hands on" practice or simulations of skills or tasks regularly performed by the healthcare professionals discussed in the chapter.

- **Critical Thinking** – Exercises that challenge you to think beyond the textbook, where answers may vary based on individual perspectives and experiences.

Contributors

Jaime Nguyen, MD, MPH, MS
Director of Allied Health Programs
Allied Health
Penn Foster, Scranton
Pennsylvania
United States

John Tomedi, BA
Freelance Writer/Editor
Howard, Pennsylvania
United States

Contents

Health Care in the United States

KNOWLEDGE CHECK

Multiple Choice

Circle the one correct answer to each of the following questions.

1. Who is credited with being the founder of nursing and making it a crucial part of the health care delivery process?
    a. Dorothea Dix.
    b. Clara Barton.
    c. Florence Nightingale.
    d. Dolly Madison.

2. Who is considered the father of modern medicine?
    a. Socrates.
    b. Hippocrates.
    c. Aristotle.
    d. Leonardo da Vinci.

3. According to historical accounts, what did the red and the white color scheme of the poles outside barber shops represent to show the availability of health care?
    a. Spirituality and togetherness.
    b. Stop and enter.
    c. Fire and water elements.
    d. Blood and bandages.

4. Personal characteristics about a given population such as age, race, and gender are considered _____ data.
    a. epidemiological.
    b. biological.
    c. demographic.
    d. objective.

5. Which health care model dictates that illness or disease requires treatment?
    a. Medical model.
    b. Wellness model.
    c. Mental health model.
    d. Provider model.

6. What is the basic idea of the wellness model?
    a. Medical treatment is a necessary service that should be free for citizens of a developed country.
    b. Disease and illness require treatment.
    c. Health is a continual process dependent on the optimal functioning of multiple aspects of a person's life.
    d. Good mental health practices dictate a person's wellbeing and help prevent physical illness.

7. What is the meaning of the term *endemic*?
    a. A sudden increase in the prevalence of a certain disease.
    b. A sudden decrease in the number of infections from a particular disease.
    c. The usual baseline level of a particular disease.
    d. The event of a disease rapidly spreading over multiple countries or continents.

8. A sudden increase in the number of reported cases for a particular disease spreading over a large geographical area is known as a(n);
    a. endemic.
    b. pandemic.
    c. epidemic.
    d. plague.

9. Which federal agency oversees the health care and public health of the United States?
   a. The Centers for Medicare and Medicaid.
   b. The Center for Disease Control.
   c. The Department of Health and Human Services.
   d. The Joint Commission.
10. In which year was the Social Security Act established, which brought both Medicare and Medicaid coverages to people of the United States?
   a. 1915.
   b. 1965.
   c. 2008.
   d. 1980.
11. Which is an example of a third-party payer?
   a. Caregiver for the patient.
   b. Family of the patient.
   c. Someone who pays by check or credit card.
   d. Health insurer.
12. Alex pays a fixed amount to his insurance company each month. This is known as the policy's
   a. premium.
   b. co-insurance.
   c. co-payment or copay.
   d. deductible.
13. Per the Affordable Care Act, insurance companies must cover individuals with _____ conditions.
   a. terminal.
   b. developmental.
   c. pre-existing.
   d. acute injury.
14. What is the common term for government health care that would pay for the medical needs of all Americans?
   a. Global health care.
   b. Universal health care.
   c. Community health care.
   d. Inclusive health care.
15. Which party funds and finances health care in a single-payer model?
   a. The patient.
   b. An insurance company.
   c. An employer.
   d. A public agency.
16. Which is a disadvantage of the single-payer model from the standpoint of a provider?
   a. A physician would likely be paid less and have no choice of insurers to work with.
   b. There would be a decrease in the patient pool.
   c. Providers would lose patients.
   d. The provider's office will have a more difficult time getting reimbursed for services rendered.
17. What is a benefit of a single-party payer for society?
   a. National expenditures on health care would decrease.
   b. Physician salaries would increase.
   c. There would be fewer and shorter wait times to see a provider.
   d. Some health insurance companies might go out of business.

True/False

Read the following statements and write "T" for true or "F" for false in the blanks provided. If a statement is false, correct the statement to make it true.
1. ____ Until the COVID-19 pandemic in 2020, there had not been a pandemic that affected the United States since the Spanish Flu pandemic of 1918.
2. ____ An example of bioterrorism is the deployment of a "dirty bomb."
3. ____ Morbidity statistics refer to the amount of disease in a population.
4. ____ Health care in the United States has shifted from the prevention and treatment of contagious diseases like tuberculosis and influenza to the prevention and treatment of diseases such as cancer, drug abuse, and heart disease.

5. ____ Since the novel COVID-19 spread over many countries and continents, it is considered an endemic.
6. ____ Health care costs are generally lower when preventative care is practiced.
7. ____ Uninsured people are less likely than those with insurance to receive preventive care and/or services for major health conditions and chronic diseases.
8. ____ The goal of the Affordable Care Act was to improve the quality of health care by compensating providers at a higher level in order to attract better and more skilled medical personnel to the field.
9. ____ Under the Affordable Care Act, children are able to stay on their parents' health care insurance policy until age 26, even if they do not live with their parents.
10. ____ Some people in countries with a single-payer system experience significant wait times for specialized care.

HEALTH CARE IN HISTORY

Historical Perspectives
Choose 10 of the milestones of health care progress from the Medical Milestones box at the end of Chapter 1 in the textbook to construct a timeline of health care progress.

```
├──────┼──────┼──────┼──────┼──────┼──────┼──────┼──────┼──────┼──────┤
      1500           1600           1700           1800           1900
```

HEALTH AND HEALTH CARE SYSTEMS

What Does Health Mean to You?
The concept of "health" has many definitions, each with a particular frame of reference. Construct a personal definition of health, one that is relevant to you.

_____

_____

_____

_____

Types of Health care Organizations
Institutional health care is provided in many different types of organizations, some offering similar services, and some with quite distinct services. Fill in the missing information in this table of health care organizations.

Provider	Services Provided
Hospice	
Public health care	
Specialty hospital	
Long-term care center	
General hospital	
Clinic	

Public Health
Public health agencies have existed for some time, but they earned a renewed prominence during the COVID-19 pandemic. Research a public health agency (it may be county, state, national, or international). Determine its purpose, along

with several services it provides. List at least three types of health care professionals who might be employed by the public health agency in your research.

Agency: _____

_____

_____

_____

_____

Purpose: _____

_____

_____

_____

_____

Services _____

_____

_____

_____

_____

Health care Professionals Employed: _____

_____

_____

_____

MEDICAL AND WELLNESS MODELS

What's Your Wellness?

The concept of health and the provision of health care in the United States have traditionally been based on the medical model, which focuses on the diagnosis and treatment of illness through standard protocols. Another model, the wellness model, has gained attention in recent years. The wellness model focuses on the prevention of disease, as well as efforts individuals can take to enjoy optimal health through attention to important aspects of life.

Box 1-2 in the textbook, Wellness Model, outlines six parameters that contribute to overall wellness. For each parameter, think of a way you can maintain or improve your functioning in that area.

Parameter	Maintain or Improve
Physical	
Intellectual	
Social	
Emotional	
Occupational	
Spiritual	

4

SINGLE-PAYER SYSTEM

Although the Affordable Care Act is sometimes confused with a single-payer system, or universal health coverage, it is not the same thing. A single-payer health system is one in which everyone has health insurance under one health insurance plan, with access to other services such as dental care and prescription medications. The plan is administered by a public agency.

Several countries have single-payer systems of health insurance, including Canada, Denmark, and Taiwan among others. As with all systems, there are pros and cons to a single-payer system. Research more about a single-payer system, and identify three advantages and three disadvantages to this form of health insurance coverage.

Advantages	Disadvantages

CRITICAL THINKING

According to the CDC, 86% of the United States' $2.7 trillion in annual health care expenditures is for chronic and mental health conditions, such as cancer, diabetes, heart disease, substance abuse, and depression.

1. What might be some of the causes of these chronic, expensive conditions?

_____

_____

_____

_____

_____

_____

2. What do you think can be done on an individual, community, governmental, and societal level to address these devastating illnesses?

_____

_____

_____

_____

_____

_____

_____

_____

3. Of those levels, which do you think is the most important to address chronic and mental health conditions? Why?

_____

_____

_____

_____

_____

_____

2 Healthcare Facilities and Organizations

KNOWLEDGE CHECK

Multiple Choice

Circle the one correct answer to each of the following questions.

1. By definition, patients at an acute care facility have an average stay of fewer than _____ days.
   a. 5
   b. 15
   c. 30
   d. 100

2. Which of these health care settings would be classified as acute inpatient care?
   a. Hospital
   b. Hospice
   c. Retail clinic
   d. Home health care

3. Hospital *privileges* allow
   a. family and friends of a patient to visit.
   b. patients to receive care at the hospital of their choice.
   c. physicians to perform procedures and admit patients to a hospital.
   d. attending physicians to take the role of a patient's PCP.

4. Which is an example of a visit or encounter?
   a. A patient is admitted to the hospital.
   b. A nursing home patient is evaluated by the nurse.
   c. A patient dies in hospice care.
   d. A patient receives care from a physician at a clinic.

5. When does a patient become an inpatient?
   a. When a provider obtains consent to treat a patient
   b. When a patient goes to the hospital
   c. When a patient goes to the emergency department
   d. When a provider writes an order to admit the patient

6. Which acute inpatient treatment setting offers psychiatric and social services to patients with mental illness?
   a. Hospice
   b. Rehabilitation hospitals
   c. Behavioral health hospitals
   d. Community centers

7. How is hospital size typically measured?
   a. Annual revenues
   b. Number of beds
   c. Length of time the facility has been open
   d. Square footage of the campus

8. Which private, nonprofit organization ensures quality of care by providing accreditation to health care facilities?
   a. Food and Drug Administration
   b. Veterans Affairs
   c. The Joint Commission
   d. The American Medical Association

9. What is the term represents the entry point for health care consumers into the health care delivery system?
   a. Tertiary care
   b. Primary care
   c. Initial care
   d. Elementary care

10. What is a *gatekeeper*?
    a. A PCP as the referrer to a specialist, such as a cardiologist, for a patient's health needs
    b. A decision-maker of an insurance claim, who will decide what services will be covered and what amount will be the fiscal responsibility of the patient
    c. An operator of a diagnostic imaging machine, especially MRI or CT scanner
    d. The third-party that allows a patient to see certain providers, either a government agency or an insurance company
11. Which type of health care setting is owned by one physician?
    a. Conglomerate
    b. Partnership
    c. Networked partnership
    d. Sole proprietorship
12. Which type of facility is designed to perform surgical procedures in a single visit?
    a. Physician's office
    b. Retail clinic
    c. Ambulatory surgery center
    d. Long-term care facility
13. What is the term for the type of treatment provided by hospice?
    a. Curative care
    b. Palliative care
    c. Mercy care
    d. Sub-acute care
14. Which of these is a long-term care (LTC) facility?
    a. Skilled nursing facility
    b. Rehabilitation hospital
    c. Assisted living facility
    d. Behavioral health hospital
15. Home health care is a form of _____ treatment for patients who are chronically ill allowing treatment in the comfort of their homes.
    a. inpatient
    b. urgent
    c. outpatient
    d. emergency
16. What is hospice care?
    a. Medical care for the terminally ill that focuses on relief of symptoms rather than cure
    b. Medical care for patients with curable ailments provided for no more than 30 days
    c. Care and housing services provided to help patients, who are often elderly, live on their own
    d. A variety services provided to patients who do no require full hospitalization, but need more than just custodial services

True/False
Read the following statements and write "T" for true or "F" for false in the blanks provided. If a statement is false, correct the statement to make it true.
1. _____ Acute care patients are inpatients.
2. _____ In general, ambulatory care services are performed in a hospital.
3. _____ A sports physical is a good example of acute care.
4. _____ A group practice is an arrangement where multiple physicians share ownership of the facility, clinic, or office.
5. _____ A *locum tenens* physician is one who serves on a temporary basis; for example, by filling in for physicians in solo practice who are unable to work for a variety of reasons.
6. _____ Urgent care clinics usually have a specialty focus, such as obstetrics and gynecology, or cardiology.
7. _____ Diagnostic facilities allow a patient to obtain tests and test results, along with treatment, if warranted, all in one location on the same day.
8. _____ Home health care services are often provided by nurses.
9. _____ Long-term care facilities are exclusively for care of older people with chronic, long-term illnesses.
10. _____ Hospice care typically includes bereavement services for the family of the terminally ill patient.

INPATIENT AND OUTPATIENT HEALTH CARE DELIVERY SETTINGS

Where Would You Go?

Health care is provided in a variety of settings. The decision about which facility to visit or type of care to seek depends on the severity of the problem at hand and the length of time treatment is expected to take (among other factors). For each of the problems listed, indicate which setting or type of care would be an appropriate choice. More than one answer may be correct.

Problem	Facility(ies) or Type of Care
Ruptured appendix	
Recovery after hip replacement	
Earache	
Stage 4 cancer with less than a 6-month expected survival rate	
Laceration requiring stitches	
Colonoscopy	

Hospitals

Hospitals are the most common type of acute care facility. In fact, hospitals are one of the largest employers in the United States, employing more than 40% of all health care workers. Not all residents of the United States live in an area served by a nearby hospital; in fact, many Americans live more than 30 minutes from the closest hospital.

Determine the hospital of each type that is closest to where you live.

Type of Hospital	Name of Closest Facility	Distance from You
General hospital		
Teaching hospital		
Specialty hospital		

Ambulatory Care

Now, do similar research as you did in the previous exercise, but identify ambulatory care settings near you and indicate a service that would be offered there.

Ambulatory Care Setting	Name of Nearby Facility	Example of Service Offered
Hospital emergency department		
Dialysis clinic		
Group practice		
Diagnostic facility		
Urgent care clinic		
Retail health clinic		

CRITICAL THINKING

Hospice Care

Hospice care provides medical care and services for people with terminal illnesses and their loved ones. Eligibility for hospice care is determined by a number of factors, one of which is a life expectancy of less than six months. Both Medicare and Medicaid provide reimbursement to some hospice care providers. While hospice care can be offered in a hospital or nursing home, it may also occur in a person's home.

Hospice care is not intended to cure the illness. It is intended to provide relief from pain, improve quality of life, and help the patient and the family plan for and process the patient's impending death.

1. The decision to enter hospice care can be a very difficult one for the person who is ill and his or her loved ones. Why do you think that is?

_____

_____

_____

_____

_____

2. What characteristics would be important for a hospice nurse to have?

_____

_____

_____

_____

_____

Different Types of Practice

The textbook discussed various types of business arrangements for physician's offices, including solo practice, group practice, and HMO ownership. Imagine that you are a physician. What do you think your preferred type of practice would be? Why?

_____

_____

_____

_____

_____

3 Healthcare Delivery and Patient Workflow

Multiple Choice

Circle the one correct answer to each of the following questions.

1. What is the term for the steps and series of processes that occur during the entire patient encounter?
   a. Admission cycle
   b. Patient portal
   c. Triage
   d. Patient workflow

2. Similar to a flowchart, a tool that helps users visualize the patient encounter process is a(n)
   a. workflow grid.
   b. workflow map.
   c. patient grid.
   d. patient processes chart.

3. What is the term for a website that can be used by patients to access their health records and do things like reschedule appointments, view lab results, and communicate with their provider?
   a. Virtual EHR
   b. Patient point of service
   c. Patient portal
   d. Virtual visit

4. The patient workflow comprises the entire patient encounter. It is divided into two main functions or processes: administrative and
   a. patient data functions.
   b. clinical functions.
   c. treatment functions.
   d. revenue functions.

5. Siddhartha is back at his physician's office for his routine check-up. He is on the schedule as a(n)
   a. new patient.
   b. established patient.
   c. annual patient.
   d. perennial patient.

6. What is the term for the process of assessing patients' conditions and prioritizing how urgently they need services?
   a. Staggering
   b. Scheduling matrix
   c. Triage
   d. Open access scheduling

7. Which categories of triage are listed from most important to least important?
   a. Non-urgent, emergent, urgent
   b. Emergent, urgent, non-urgent
   c. Urgent, non-urgent, emergent
   d. Urgent, emergent, non-urgent

8. What is another term for fixed appointment scheduling, which assigns patients into specific time blocks of 15- to 30-minute increments - sometimes longer for new patients?
   a. Staggered schedule
   b. Wave scheduling
   c. Stream scheduling
   d. Modified wave scheduling

9. Which scheduling technique schedules a group of patients at the beginning of an hour who are then seen in the order in which they arrive?
   a. Wave
   b. Staggered
   c. Streaming
   d. Open access

10. What is the short amount of time, about 15 minutes, right before the provider actually sees the patient?
   a. Preauthorized minutes
   b. Common time
   c. Lead time
   d. Pre-visit minutes

11. What is open access scheduling?
   a. A scheduling technique used when there is an increase in patient flow
   b. A scheduling technique used when there is a decrease in patient flow
   c. A type of scheduling that allows for patients to schedule their own appointments by using the patient portal
   d. A scheduling technique that allows patients to be seen as they arrive, without appointments

12. What is the most commonly used appointment scheduling system?
   a. Wave scheduling
   b. Open access scheduling
   c. Stream scheduling
   d. Wave scheduling

13. Which scheduling system lowers the chance of a provider having to wait for a patient who arrives late?
   a. Double booking
   b. Staggered scheduling
   c. Stream scheduling
   d. Wave scheduling

14. What is double booking?
   a. When two patients are scheduled for the same time slot of the same provider
   b. When a redundant procedure, such as a lab, is set to happen for the same patient by accident
   c. When one patient is scheduled with two providers at the same time
   d. When the scheduler puts the patient down for multiple appointments

15. Which type of scheduling involves putting patient with similar needs on the schedule together?
   a. Similar scheduling
   b. Group scheduling
   c. Cluster scheduling
   d. Support scheduling

16. Which part of the "SOAP" technique represents the patient's view of the presenting problem?
   a. Subjective
   b. Objective
   c. Assessment
   d. Plan

17. During the clinical assessment, patients are asked about their reason for seeking medical care, also known as the
   a. central problem.
   b. chief complaint.
   c. chief concern.
   d. grand issue.

18. Which of these is not performed at patient checkout?
   a. Discharge instructions are given.
   b. Follow-up appointments are made.
   c. The patient pays the fee for service or copay.
   d. Insurance is verified.

True or False

Read the following statements and write "T" for true or "F" for false in the blanks provided. If a statement is false, correct the statement to make it true.

1. _____ An efficient and effective clinical workflow's primary purpose is to improve the healthcare facility's finances.

2. ____ Patient workflow can be defined as a series of steps that personnel in a healthcare facility take in order to assess and manage patient care.

3. ____ For all intents and purposes, the patient workflow for an inpatient setting is pretty much the same as for an outpatient setting.

4. ____ Triage occurs exclusively in the emergency department setting.

5. ____ A patient who has had a prior admission to a hospital will be considered an established patient should he or she be admitted in the future, and any information obtained during the new visit will be added to the patient's existing account number.

6. ____ The healthcare professional who performs triage in an emergency department is typically a nurse.

7. ____ The most flexible type of scheduling is stream scheduling.

8. ____ Walk-in patients should arrive 15 minutes before their appointment - 30 minutes before for new patients.

9. ____ In 2007, the Centers for Medicare and Medicaid Services (CMS) began prohibiting providers from charging fees for missed appointments.

10. ____ Melanie needs to see both a physical therapist and an occupational therapist. She is scheduled for these providers on the same date and time, a technique called double booking.

11. ____ Information collected during the patient registration process includes height, weight, and vital signs.

12. ____ A symptom is subjective and experienced by the patient, while a sign is objective can be observed by the clinician.

13. ____ A common method of documenting the medical evaluation and treatment plan is by using SOAP notes.

PATIENT WORKFLOW

The Steps in Patient Workflow

Order the following steps for a physician's office patient workflow.

a. _____ Dr Lane's medical assistant takes Larissa's temperature, heart rate, and blood pressure, and asks what brings her in today.

b. _____ Dr Lane's receptionist schedules an appointment for the following afternoon at 2 pm, and asks Larissa to arrive at 1:45 pm.

c. _____ Larissa arrives at Dr Lane's office at 1:50 pm and completes several forms requesting her updated health status and release of information for billing, per HIPAA. She provides her current insurance information.

d. _____ Dr Lane examines Larissa's arm and asks her questions about her recent exposure to any irritants, such as plants, animals, or new lotions, fabrics, or laundry detergent.

e. _____ Larissa schedules a follow-up appointment with Dr Lane for 4 weeks from today.

f. _____ Larissa Jenkins notices a rash on her arm. She calls her regular primary care provider, Dr Lane.

g. _____ Dr Lane's administrative staff verify Larissa's insurance.

Inpatient vs Outpatient Clinical Workflow

Indicate whether each action is more likely to occur in an inpatient (I) or an outpatient (O) setting, or equally likely to occur in both (B).

1. _____ The patient makes an appointment for his annual physical examination via the patient portal.

2. _____ The patient's height and weight are recorded.

3. _____ The patient complains of chest pain, and after performing an EKG, the physician orders an ambulance to transfer the patient to the nearest ED.

4. _____ The patient is discharged to a skilled nursing facility after repair of a broken hip.

5. _____ The patient's insurance information is collected.

6. _____ The scheduler chooses a 60-minute appointment slot for a new patient visit.

7. _____ The patient waits in the waiting room.

8. _____ A physician performs a physical examination.

9. _____ Nurses monitor and care for the patient for two nights.

Evaluation of the Workflow

Workflows should be evaluated on a regular basis to ensure that they remain efficient and effective. How might the following changes affect a clinical workflow?

1. The physician hires a nurse practitioner to see patients who request appointments for acute minor ailments and maintenance of chronic conditions, while the physician handles annual physical exams.

2. The practice manager decides to buy X-ray equipment in order to obtain X-rays in-house, without having to refer patients to imaging centers.

3. Timco Insurance, a third-party payer that insures many of the clinic's patients, changes its requirements. Its enrolled patients now need to obtain precertification before a referral to a specialist can be made.

4. New regulations require that all patients receiving Medicaid be asked if they want a flu shot during any visit to a doctor, and that their response be recorded in their EHR. If the response is positive, a flu shot must be provided during that visit.

5. Now it's your turn; describe a situation that would create the need for change in the clinical workflow:

_____

_____

_____

_____

_____

SCHEDULING

Scheduling Method Pros and Cons

For each scheduling method, describe at least one potential advantage and disadvantage for the healthcare provider and facility using it. Then look at it from the patients' viewpoint, and described a potential advantage and disadvantage for them.

1. Stream Scheduling
   a. Provider Advantage

   _____

   _____

   b. Provider Disadvantage

   _____

   _____

   a. Patient Advantage

   _____

   _____

   b. Patient Disadvantage

   _____

   _____

2. Wave Scheduling
   a. Provider Advantage

   _____

   _____

b. Provider Disadvantage

_____

_____

_____

a. Patient Advantage

_____

_____

_____

b. Patient Disadvantage

_____

_____

_____

3. Staggered Scheduling
   a. Provider Advantage

_____

_____

_____

b. Provider Disadvantage

_____

_____

_____

a. Patient Advantage

_____

_____

_____

b. Patient Disadvantage

_____

_____

_____

Types of Patient Encounters in a Medical Office

Different types of patient encounters require different administrative tasks and different clinical assessments. Give an example of the reason a patient might schedule each type of appointment. Would a complete patient registration occur, or would the patient's current information be updated for the visit?

An example is provided.

Type of Visit	Possible Reason	New Registration, Update, or Depends
Follow-up visit	A patient returns to the referring doctor after undergoing physical therapy for a torn tendon	Update
New patient		
Well-child visit		
Urgent visit		
Phone encounter		

The SOAP Note

A common method of documenting the medical evaluation and treatment plan is by using a SOAP note. Indicate which part of the SOAP note each piece of information belongs in.

S: Patient's Subjective View
O: Provider's Objective View
A: Provider's Assessment
P: Treatment Plan

1. _____ Patient to return for re-evaluation in 2 weeks.
2. _____ Patient states he's been waking up because his throat hurts so much.
3. _____ Patient's temperature is 101°F
4. _____ Patient has pharyngitis (sore throat).
5. _____ Antibiotics prescribed for 14 days.
6. _____ Patient's throat is red and patchy upon examination using a pen light.
7. _____ Patient reports feeling feverish for 48 hours.

Sign or Symptom?

The words sign and symptom are often used interchangeably in everyday language. However, in clinical terms, they have different meanings. A sign is an objective, measurable indicator of disease. A symptom is a subjective indicator of disease experienced by the patient.

Indicate whether each indicator is a sign or a symptom.

Indicator	Sign or Symptom?
Foot pain	
Blisters	
Headache	
Fatigue	
Weight change	
Trouble hearing	
Nasal discharge	

CRITICAL THINKING

In this chapter, you have learned about the importance of an effective and efficient workflow in the operation of a health-care facility. It's not just facilities that benefit from the use of workflow management strategies; individuals do as well. What does your personal workflow look like for a day? Write it out or create a workflow map, as in Figure 3-1 of the textbook. As you review your workflow, consider whether there are any changes you would like to make to improve your personal effectiveness and efficiency.

_____

_____

_____

_____

_____

_____

4 Healthcare Workforce

KNOWLEDGE CHECK

Multiple Choice

1. Which is a requirement of the state government for professionals in certain industries to practice?
   a. License
   b. Registration
   c. Credential
   d. Professional credential

2. In healthcare, which is true of registration and licensing?
   a. Licensing is easy to sign up for and obtain, but expensive.
   b. Registration with a professional medical organization gives the ability to practice under law, whereas a license is more of a membership.
   c. Licensing is permission from the state medical board allowing the legal practice of medicine.
   d. Registration is mandatory and expected by employers.

3. The letters that follow Paula's name, Paula Wilska, RN, are known as
   a. licensees.
   b. acronyms.
   c. credentials.
   d. registrars.

4. A doctor who has completed training at a school that is focused primarily on manipulation of the spinal column is known as a(n)
   a. DC.
   b. DO.
   c. MD.
   d. APRN.

5. What is an allied health professional?
   a. A physician in a network that shares electronic health records
   b. An individual who complements and assists the work of physicians and other healthcare providers
   c. Any healthcare employee licensed to practice in his or her state
   d. A participating primary care provider in a large healthcare system, such as an HMO

6. The Health Sciences Career Cluster of allied health professionals includes all categories except
   a. therapeutic services.
   b. surgical procedures.
   c. research and development.
   d. health informatics.

7. Which is **not** a skill set covered under the National Career Clusters Framework for allied health professionals?
   a. Health promotion
   b. Treatment of injuries and diseases
   c. Physical examination and diagnosis
   d. Wellness and diagnosis

8. According to the Association of Schools of Allied Health Professions, how much of the healthcare workforce is composed of allied health professionals?
   a. About 25%
   b. About 10%
   c. About 95%
   d. About 60%

9. Which credential might be held by a nurse whose education was a 2-year degree?
   a. LPN
   b. APRN
   c. PA
   d. CMA
10. Which credential is offered by the Federation of State Medical Boards or the National Board of Medical Examiners?
    a. DO
    b. MD
    c. RN
    d. ARPN
11. There are many paths to careers in healthcare. In almost all cases, a _____ is required to get started.
    a. high school diploma or equivalent
    b. training in a vocation
    c. medical degree
    d. technical training
12. What is the meaning of the term *stakeholder* as it relates to a business or healthcare clinic?
    a. One who is registered with a professional organization
    b. One who holds the proper credentials in their professional field
    c. One with an interest related to the operations of the organization
    d. One who is at the top of the executive flow chart
13. Medical billers and coders do not require a _____ to legally practice, but typically hold a _____.
    a. credential, license
    b. license, credential
    c. registration, license
    d. credential, registration
14. Tanisha is a nurse in the emergency of the local hospital. She has the authority and responsibility to give the patient medications, but she is not allowed to prescribe medications based on her understanding of the patient's condition. The term for this limitation is called
    a. realm of responsibility.
    b. scope of practice.
    c. responsibility reach.
    d. provisions of workplace.
15. Which part of the healthcare delivery process involves diagnosing and treating patients?
    a. Administrative
    b. Coding
    c. Clinical
    d. Management

True/False

Read the following statements and write "T" for true or "F" for false in the blanks provided. If a statement is false, correct the statement to make it true.
1. _____ Licensing is desired, but not required, for a physician to practice.
2. _____ The provider agency of the credential for Doctor of Osteopathy (DO) is the National Board of Medical Examiners (NBME).
3. _____ Almost all healthcare professionals will have some type of certification.
4. _____ Only professionals in a healthcare setting, such as a hospital or clinic, are addressed as "doctor."
5. _____ MDs and DOs are both licensed physicians, equally qualified to practice medicine.
6. _____ The purpose of a medical treatment plan is to guide other providers involved in the treatment of the patient.
7. _____ The career title of "technologist" typically requires some classroom and clinical preparation OR on-the-job training.
8. _____ The national non-profit organization that created the National Career Clusters Framework is the Career and Technology Education (CTE).

CREDENTIALING, LICENSING, AND REGISTRATION

Education Requirements

Provide the missing information in the table.

Professional	Educational Requirement	Diploma/Degree	Example
Assistant			
Technician			
Professional			
Aide			
Technologist			

Understanding the Concepts

In your own words, explain registration, credentialing, and licensing, and provide an example of a healthcare professional who would receive that designation.

1. Registration:

_____

_____

_____

2. Credential:

_____

_____

_____

3. License:

_____

_____

_____

Different Doctors

Write out the full name of the type of doctor for which each abbreviation is used.

1. Ed.D. _____

2. D.O. _____

3. Ph.D. _____

4. D.C. _____

5. D.M.D. _____

6. N.D. _____

7. D.D.S. _____

8. D.P.M. _____

ALLIED HEALTH PROFESSIONALS

Allied or Medical Health Professional

Indicate whether each job title is for an allied health professional or medical health professional. Remember that allied health professionals assist, facilitate, or complement the work of medical health professionals, such as doctors.

1. Medical coder_____
2. Registered nurse_____
3. Pharmacy technician_____
4. Physical therapist_____
5. Physician_____
6. Surgical technician_____
7. Dentist_____
8. Phlebotomist_____
9. Biochemist_____
10. Diagnostic imaging technician_____

Researching Allied Health and Medical Health Careers

Choose an allied health profession and a medical health profession to research. Find out and record information for each in the chart below.

The textbook includes websites that might be helpful in the "Explore the Web" section, and the — Bureau of Labor Statistics maintains an Occupational Outlook Handbook online that is easily searchable (https://www.bls.gov/ooh/).

Allied Health Profession: _____	Education/Training Requirements	
	Job Duties	
	Salary Range	
Medical Health Profession: _____	Education/Training Requirements	
	Job Duties	
	Salary Range	

CRITICAL THINKING

Expanding the Scope of Practice

The United States is currently facing a shortage of both physicians and nurses. In response, several states have passed legislation allowing other healthcare professionals to perform some duties traditionally reserved for physicians. For example, in some states, physician assistants may provide care without a physician being present, and nurse practitioners can practice without physician oversight. Proponents of expanding the scope of practice argue that these healthcare professionals can be trained and licensed more quickly and less expensively than physicians can, and they can practice without compromising safety and quality. However, some physicians' groups disagree, arguing that their more intensive and extensive training better equips them to diagnose more accurately and provide patient care more safely.

1. What is your opinion of enabling non-physician medical providers to provide medical care and procedures that have traditionally been reserved for physicians? Please explain your position.

_____

_____

_____

_____

_____

_____

_____

_____

_____

Naturopathic Medical Doctors

A naturopathic medical doctor (ND or NMD) focuses on holistic and preventative healthcare. A naturopathic doctor is a licensed primary care physician, who is trained to diagnose and prescribe treatment, as with other physicians, but emphasizes naturopathic medicine and the use of natural healing agents, such as food, herbs, and water. However, many states do not regulate naturopathic medicine as a medical profession.

1. Why do you think some states do not license naturopathic medical doctors?

_____

_____

_____

_____

_____

_____

_____

_____

2. Do you think licensing naturopathic medical doctors is a good idea? Why or why not?

_____

_____

_____

_____

_____

_____

_____

_____

5 Healthcare Law and Ethics

KNOWLEDGE CHECK

Multiple Choice

1. What is the meaning of the concept of *respondeat superior*?
   a. The customer is always right.
   b. The employees of a company are responsible for their behavior.
   c. An employer is liable for the actions of its employees.
   d. Companies must respond to complaints quickly.

2. What is the term for a private and civil wrong that causes an injury?
   a. Negligence
   b. Living will
   c. Tort
   d. Jurisprudent

3. Mrs Morris is 88 years old and has been admitted to the hospital. She asks if she may decide which type of care is offered in the event she cannot communicate. Which document(s) should be provided to her?
   a. Power of attorney
   b. Advance directives
   c. Last will and testament
   d. Waiver of additional care form

4. Which act of improper activity or treatment is determined by a negative answer to the question, "Would a similarly skilled healthcare professional have provided the same treatment under the same circumstances?"
   a. Battery
   b. Assault
   c. Abandonment
   d. Malpractice

5. Which offense is proved by four basic elements: duty of care, dereliction of duty, direct cause, and damages?
   a. Assault
   b. Negligence
   c. Malpractice
   d. Abandonment

6. What is the name for the party who brings a legal action to court?
   a. Plaintiff
   b. Solicitor
   c. Defendant
   d. Adjudicator

7. Which laws protect the rights of the state or government?
   a. Criminal law
   b. Civil law
   c. Medical law
   d. Mediation

8. Someone who commits a felony is guilty of violating which kind of law?
   a. Civil law
   b. Medical law
   c. Criminal law
   d. State statutes

9. Joey vandalized an old building and was charged with a misdemeanor. Assuming it is Joey's first offense, this type of crime is usually punishable by
   a. imprisonment.
   b. monetary fines.

23

c. trial by jury.

d. a felony charge on his criminal record.

10. Which crime can occur when a procedure is performed on a patient without consent?
    a. Assault
    b. Battery
    c. Negligence
    d. Malpractice

11. A healthcare worker must be _____, meaning they are aware of the laws that impact the healthcare industry.
    a. liable
    b. jurisprudent
    c. *respondeat superior*
    d. tort

12. Workers in all occupations, including healthcare, are legally _____ for their actions.
    a. jurisprudent
    b. *respondeat superior*
    c. liable
    d. maleficent

13. Healthcare professionals must stay within a scope of practice and only use methods for which they have been trained. For example, Manny is a nurse and, by law, offers care under his state's
    a. Nursing Protection Act (NPA).
    b. Nurse Procedure Act (NPA).
    c. Nurse Practice Act (NPA).
    d. National Practice Act (NPA).

14. Based on experience, religion, and philosophy, _____ in healthcare are the basis of behavior that gives respect for the needs and rights of others.
    a. morals
    b. ethics
    c. rights
    d. statutes

15. The first code of ethics for the medical profession is the
    a. Code of Hammurabi.
    b. Vaidya's Oath.
    c. Hippocratic Oath.
    d. ABIM physician charter.

16. What is necessary in order for the patient to feel comfortable enough to share vital and personal information with the provider?
    a. Bedside manner
    b. Confidentiality
    c. Hippocratic Oath
    d. Jurisprudence

17. To ensure patient privacy and try to reduce administrative costs of healthcare, _____ was passed in 1996 by Congress.
    a. the Hill-Burton Act (HBA)
    b. the National Labor Relations Act (NLRA)
    c. the Health Insurance Portability and Accountability Act (HIPAA)
    d. the National Medical Care Expenditure Act (NMCEA)

18. Most healthcare entities have constructed some type of guidelines or policies to ensure the protection and safety of patients. In 1973, the American Hospital Association (AHA) adopted the _____, which was revised in 1992.
    a. Provider and Patient Security Standards
    b. Patients' Bill of Rights
    c. Health Insurance Portability and Accountability Act (HIPAA)
    d. Protected Health Information Doctrine

19. If protected health information (PHI) is released or sold for personal gain or malicious harm, the criminal penalties can be up to
    a. $25,000 and 5 years in prison.
    b. $250,000 and 10 years in prison.
    c. $25,000 and 5 years in prison.
    d. $250,000 and 1 year in prison.

20. Which healthcare document is **not** a type of advance directive?
    a. Living will
    b. Informed consent
    c. Power of attorney
    d. Do-not-resuscitate order

21. Which healthcare document allows another person to make medical decisions if the patient is unable to do so themselves?
    a. Do-not-resuscitate (DNR) order
    b. *living* will
    c. Durable power of attorney
    d. Last will and testament

22. Organ donation is controlled at the _____ level and is regulated by the 1968 National Organ Transplant Act.
    a. state
    b. county
    c. national
    d. global

HEALTHCARE LAW

Fill in the Blank

Fill in each of the spaces provided with the missing word or words that complete the sentence.

1. Generally speaking, there are two main categories of law: _____ and _____ _____.

2. Violations of _____ law are called crimes, which include _____ _____, lesser crimes often punishable by state-established monetary fines or imprisonment up to a year).

3. The legal term for the threat of bodily harm that causes fear in the victim is called _____.

4. _____ laws are those that protect the private rights of a person or a person's property.

5. The most common tort against healthcare professionals is for _____.

6. An act of negligence that involves an improper or illegal professional activity or treatment is termed _____ _____.

7. The individual with the _____ license, training, or authority in an organization is usually the one ultimately responsible for the actions of his or her employees.

In the News

Find and read an article that describes a current legal or ethical case relating to the healthcare industry. Then answer the following questions.

1. Title of article:_____

2. Source:_____

3. Date of publication:_____

4. What is the legal breach or issue in dispute in the case described in the article?

_____
_____
_____
_____
_____

5. Summarize the plaintiff's point of view in the case.

_____

_____

_____

_____

_____

6. Summarize the defendant's point of view in the case.

_____

_____

_____

_____

_____

PROFESSIONAL CODE OF CONDUCT, ETHICS, AND MORALS

Scope of Practice

Use the Internet to research the scope of practice of a nurse assistant, registered nurse, or other health care practitioner. Prepare a presentation that describes the findings. Discuss the scope of practice of the occupation with class members as directed by your instructor.

Classifying Conduct

In the following situations, identify whether a legal or ethical breach of conduct is described. Circle the word that corresponds to your choice. If the breach is a legal consideration, explain which crime has occurred.

1. A patient in the hospital is angry about her care. She rings her bell 10 or more times an hour. You decide that she is just seeking attention, and you ignore the bell.
   Legal or Ethical Explanation:

   _____

   _____

   _____

   _____

   _____

2. You are helping a nurse who is changing a dressing on a patient's wound, and you drop the sterile dressing on the floor. You know that no one saw the dressing drop, and you replace it on the sterile tray to save time and avoid getting into trouble.
   Legal or Ethical Explanation:

   _____

   _____

   _____

   _____

   _____

3. On arriving home, you find that you have accidentally taken a pen and a roll of tape from work. You decide they are not worth returning and place them in your drawer for use at home.
   Legal or Ethical Explanation:

   _____

   _____

   _____

   _____

   _____

4. You tell your best friend that, in your role as a student healthcare worker, you saw a student from your school admitted to the hospital because of an overdose. You name the student who was admitted, and your friend promises not to tell anyone else about it. Your friend does not tell anyone.
   Legal or Ethical Explanation:

   _____

   _____

   _____

   _____

   _____

5. You observe a family in the emergency department after an accident in which one of the children was injured. The family acts very dramatically by crying and clinging to the hospital staff. You mimic that family's reaction for your friends during the football game that evening.

Legal or Ethical Explanation:

_____

_____

_____

_____

_____

Understanding HIPAA

Design a pamphlet explaining the content of the HIPAA Privacy Rule or Security Rule. Be prepared to use the pamphlet to explain the law to the class as directed by the instructor.

PATIENTS' RIGHTS

Thinking About Patient Rights

Imagine that you or someone you love has been admitted to the hospital from the emergency department. Review Box 5-6, Patient's Bill of Rights, in the textbook. Think of an example of a healthcare worker honoring the rights listed in that box, and an example of a healthcare worker ignoring those rights.

1. The right to respectful care

_____

_____

_____

_____

_____

2. The right to receive current, relevant, and understandable information

_____

_____

_____

_____

_____

3. The right to know the identity of everyone involved in their care

_____

_____

_____

_____

_____

4. The right to make decisions about the plan of care prior to undergoing treatment

_____

_____

_____

_____

_____

5. The right to privacy

_____

_____

_____

_____

_____

Informed Consent

Examine the sample consent form in Figure 5-1. Using Box 5-7 of the textbook, Elements of Informed Consent, indicate the sections in Figure 5-1 that correspond to each numbered element described in Box 5-7.

Community Hospital
555 Street Drive
Town, NJ 07999
(973) 555-5555

554879
Green, John
44 Avenue Street
Town, NJ 07999

Dr. Ramundo

Consent to Operation or Other Procedure(s)

1. I understand that _____ is proposed to be performed by _____ and/or his/her associates and whomever may be designated as assistants.

2. I understand that the nature and purpose of the operation or procedure is to _____ _____ _____

3. I understand that possible alternative methods of treatment are _____ _____ _____

4. I understand that the risks and possible complications of this operation or procedure are _____ _____

5. I am aware that the practice of medicine and surgery is not an exact science and I acknowledge that no guarantees have been made to me as to the result of this procedure.

6. I consent to the examination and disposition by hospital authorities of any tissue or parts which may be removed during the course of this operation or procedure.

7. I understand the nature of the proposed operation or procedure(s), the risks and possible complications involved, and the expected results, as described above, and hereby request that such operation or procedure(s) be performed.

8. I realize that an operation or procedure requires numerous assistants, technicians, nurses, and other personnel and I give my consent to care by such personnel before, during, and after the operation or procedure to be performed.

9. I also consent to videotaping or photographing of the operation or procedure for scientific or teaching purposes.

Witness (may not be a member of operating team)   Date

Interpreter   Date

Signature of patient, agent, or legal guardian   Date

I have discussed with the above patient the nature of the proposed operation or procedure(s), the risks and possible complications involved, and the expected results, as described above.

Signature of counseling physician

Figure 5-1 Sample consent form. From Davis, N: *Foundations of health information management*, ed 5, St. Louis, 2020, Elsevier.

Advance Directives

Advance directives are often considered concerns primarily for older individuals and/or those with terminal illnesses. That is understandable, given the greater incidence of morbidity and mortality in those populations. However, thinking about our own wishes for care should we become terminally ill or unresponsive, and how we want our remains to be handled, is something we might consider at any point in our lives.

Using Box 5-8, Elements of the Advance Directives, in the textbook, consider your positions on each of the following questions.

1. If you were able to name your own healthcare agent, who would it be? Who would be the second person in case the first person was unavailable? Why?

   _____

   _____

   _____

2. If you incurred injuries that resulted in your being in a medically diagnosed permanent vegetative state, what would your preferences be regarding your care, specifically whether you'd want:

   CPR in the case of cardiac arrest_____

   Mechanical ventilation_____

   Tube feeding_____

   Dialysis_____

   Antibiotics or antiviral medications_____

   Comfort care (e.g., avoiding invasive tests, pain medications, being allowed to die at home)

   _____

   Organ and tissue donation_____

   Body donation_____

3. What factors influenced your decision-making about these questions?

   _____

   _____

   _____

   _____

CRITICAL THINKING

In January 2009, Nadya Suleman gave birth to octuplets as a result of in vitro fertilization. This event caused a great deal of controversy over the ethical decision-making of Dr Michael Kamrava, her fertility specialist. At the time of Ms Suleman's in vitro fertilization that resulted in the birth of octuplets, she was unemployed and had six children, all from in vitro fertilization. Implanting multiple embryos can be risky, but Ms Suleman completed an informed consent. The hospital cost was estimated to be $2 million.

Dr Kamrava himself stated that the decision to implant the embryos was based on his love of children, his desire not to discard Ms Suleman's existing embryos, the informed consent of Ms Suleman, and his personal value of choice.

Was Dr Kamrava wrong to perform the procedure? Explain the ethics of your answer.

_____

_____

_____

_____

_____

_____

_____

_____

_____

29

_____

_____

_____

_____

_____

6 Medical Terminology and Body Systems

KNOWLEDGE CHECK

Multiple Choice

1. A medical terms that is made up of the first letter of each word, such as COPD is called a(n)
   a. abbreviation.
   b. acronym.
   c. prefix.
   d. eponym.

2. A word or phrase in the front of a medical term to indicate location, time, or amount is known as a(n)
   a. eponym.
   b. word root.
   c. suffix.
   d. prefix.

3. Medical terms that can be broken down into parts to determine their meaning are referred to as
   a. catalysts.
   b. breakable.
   c. decodable.
   d. simplifiers.

4. Parkinson disease is an example of which type of medical term?
   a. An acronym
   b. A proper form
   c. An eponym
   d. A root word

5. What is the meaning of the word root "ot/"?
   a. Olfactory
   b. Bone
   c. Ear
   d. Eye

6. The abbreviation RBC stands for
   a. rapid bilateral condition.
   b. recurring body conditions.
   c. red blood cell.
   d. random blood collection.

7. Blood is a type of _____ tissue.
   a. muscle
   b. epithelial
   c. nervous
   d. connective

8. Body systems consist of _____ that work together to provide a major body function.
   a. tissues
   b. cells
   c. muscles
   d. organs

9. What is the study of body structures and their location?
   a. Biology
   b. Anthropology
   c. Anatomy
   d. Physiology

31

10. Which type of tissue is made of protein fibers and has the unique property of shortening in length to produce movement?
    a. Muscle tissue
    b. Epithelial tissue
    c. Nervous tissue
    d. Connective tissue

11. Which body plane separates the front and back of the body?
    a. Sagittal
    b. Coronal
    c. Superior
    d. Transverse

12. An organ or growth above the transverse plane is referred to as
    a. inferior.
    b. superior.
    c. distal.
    d. medial.

13. The integumentary system is made up of the skin and hair, nails, specialized glands, and nerves. What is the term for the parts other than the skin?
    a. Auxiliary structures
    b. Alternative structures
    c. Accessory structures
    d. Ancillary structures

14. The _____ is a double membrane that covers the outside of the heart, providing lubrication between the heart and surrounding structures to prevent tissue damage.
    a. endocardium
    b. peritoneum
    c. endometrium
    d. pericardium

15. Apocrine and eccrine glands in the skin produce
    a. semen.
    b. sweat.
    c. tears.
    d. sebum.

16. One function of the cardiovascular system is to transport nutrients and _____ to the cells of the body.
    a. minerals
    b. vitamins
    c. oxygen
    d. hemoglobin

17. The human heart beats how many times per day?
    a. Between 10,000 and 20,000
    b. Between 25,000 and 40,000
    c. Between 60,000 and 80,000
    d. Between 85,000 and 150,000

18. What are the lower chambers of the heart called?
    a. Atria
    b. Ventricles
    c. Septum
    d. Semilunar

19. Gases, nutrients, and wastes are exchanged through the walls of tiny vessels called _____.
    a. arteries
    b. veins
    c. capillaries
    d. aorta

20. Lymph is located in all body tissues except the brain and the
    a. placenta.
    b. spinal cord.

c. ovaries.

d. testicles.

True/False

Read the following statements and write "T" for true or "F" for false in the blanks provided. If a statement is false, correct the statement to make it true.

_____ 1. Blood consists of four parts: red blood cells, white blood cells, platelets, and water.

_____ 2. Another word for white blood cells (WBCs) is leukocytes.

_____ 3. Each red blood cell (RBC) lives 1-3 days.

_____ 4. The function of the lymphatic system is to produce hormones.

_____ 5. There are two processes of respiration: external (bringing oxygen into the lungs) and internal (the exchange of oxygen and carbon dioxide).

_____ 6. The diaphragm contracts and moves downward during inhalation. This creates a suction pulling air in from outside the body.

_____ 7. The adult human body has more than 300 bones.

_____ 8. Red marrow makes blood cells for the body and also destroys old red blood cells.

_____ 9. Skeletal muscle makes up more than 40% of a person's body weight.

_____ 10. The digestive tract is about 5 feet long.

_____ 11. The wave-like contractions that push waste and food through the intestines, as well as urine from the kidneys to the bladder, is called peristalsis.

_____ 12. The thymus produces insulin and glucagon.

_____ 13. There are separate spinal nerves for motor functions and sensory functions.

MEDICAL TERMINOLOGY

Matching

Match the numbered term below with its best definition.

a. Medical term that has been shortened for convenience

b. Word formed from the first letter of each of a set of words in phrase

c. Word root with a combining vowel to enhance pronunciation

d. Medical word that can be broken down into Latin or Greek word parts to determine the meaning

e. A disease, condition, or procedure named for a person

f. Medical term that cannot be broken down into language source parts to determine the meaning

g. A phrase placed at the beginning of a medical term to indicate a location, time, or amount

h. Phrase placed at the end of a medical term to modify or change its meaning indicating a disease, procedure, or condition

i. Character or image that is used to represent something else

j. Central part of a medical term that is often derived from a Latin or Greek language source

1.	Word root
2.	Eponym
3.	Prefix
4.	Suffix
5.	Nondecodable term
6.	Decodable term
7.	Symbol
8.	Abbreviation

9.	Acronym		
10.	Combining form		

Using Prefixes, Roots, and Suffixes

Complete the following table, supplying the missing word part, word, or meaning.

Use the following prefixes, roots, and suffixes to make and define medical terms.

Word Part	Word Part	Word	Meaning
lapar/o	-tomy		Incision into the abdomen
	-ectomy	pneumonectomy	Removal of the lung
hem/o	-gram		
thorac/o			Incision into the chest
	-itis		Inflammation of a blood clot
path/o		*pathologu*	The study of disease
pept/o	-ic		
ot/o	-itis		
tympan/o		tympanitis	

BODY STRUCTURE AND ORGANIZATION

Identifying Body Planes

Identify the body planes in the images below.

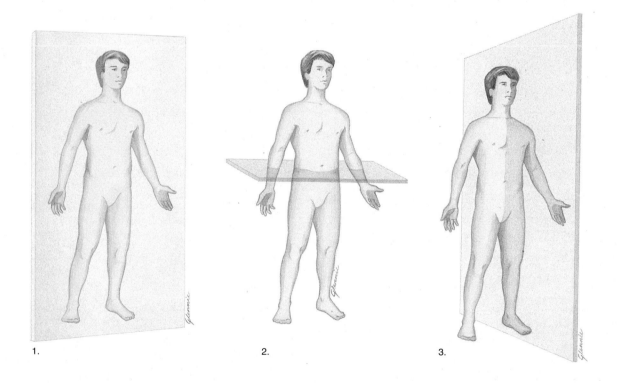

1.   2.   3.

1. _____
2. _____
3. _____

Identifying Body Cavities

Identify the body cavities in the images below.

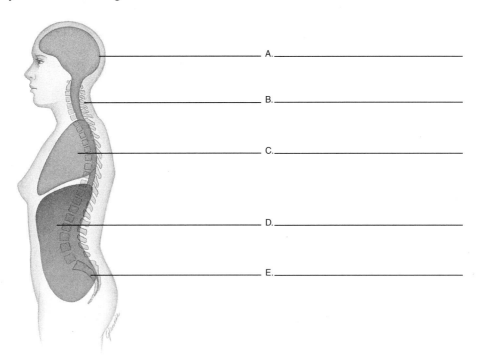

A. _____
B. _____
C. _____
D. _____
E. _____

Identifying Body Regions

Identify the body regions in the image below.

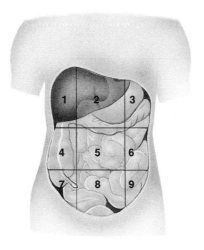

1. _____

2. _____

3. _____

4. _____

5. _____

6. _____

7. _____

8. _____

9. _____

BODY SYSTEMS

Identifying System Functions

For each function in the left column, indicate which system performs it, and provide the name of one organ or structure involved in that system.

Function	System	Organ or Structure
Helps remove wastes, supports immune system		
Regulates the environment and directs the activities of the other body systems		
Exchanges gases between the air and blood		
Transports oxygen and nutrients to all body parts and removes wastes		
Covers the body and protects other body systems		
Provides for human reproduction		
Coordinates body activities through hormones		
Provides body support and protection		
Allows the body to move and controls movements within the body		
Processes food and eliminates food waste		
Filters the blood and removes liquid wastes		

INTEGUMENTARY SYSTEM

Identifying Skin Layers

Identify the labeled skin layers and different structures in the image below.

A. _____

B. _____

C. _____

D. _____

E. _____

F. _____

G. _____

H. _____

I. _____

J. _____

K. _____

L. _____

CARDIOVASCULAR SYSTEM

Fill in the Blank

Fill in each of the spaces provided with the missing word or words that complete the sentence.

1. The _____ side of the heart pumps deoxygenated blood to the lungs.

2. _____ circulation is the path of blood from the intestines, gallbladder, pancreas, stomach, and spleen through the liver.

3. The heart has four chambers. The top chambers are called _____, and the bottom chambers are called _____.

4. Four _____ prevent blood from flowing backward through the heart.

5. The heart has _____ types of tissue.

6. The _____ layer of the heart pumps blood through the system.

7. The activity of the heart muscle is controlled mainly by the _____ system.
8. The "pacemaker" that starts a heart contraction is a collection of specialized _____ cells in the right atrium.
9. With the exception of the _____, blood in the arteries is oxygenated.
10. Blood has four components: red blood cells, white blood cells, _____, and plasma.
11. Red blood cells contain a protein called _____ that carries oxygen to all cells and removes carbon dioxide.
12. _____ are a type of white blood cell that help defend the body from allergic reactions and parasitic infections.
13. _____ are the smallest type of blood cell.
14. Every second, a few million new red blood cells are made in a process called _____.

The Movement of Blood Through the Heart

Complete the missing information in the table below.

Structure	Oxygenated or Deoxygenated	Blood Goes From Here to The...
Body	Both	Inferior and superior vena cavae
Inferior and superior vena cavae		Right atrium
Right atrium		
	Deoxygenated	
	Deoxygenated	Pulmonary valve
	Deoxygenated	Pulmonary artery
	Deoxygenated	
	Both	
		Left atrium
Left atrium		
	Oxygenated	
		Aortic valve
Aortic valve		
		Body

LYMPHATIC SYSTEM

Lymphatic System Fill in the Blank

Fill in each of the spaces provided with the missing word or words that complete the sentence.
1. The lymphatic system works with the _____ system to return body fluids to the blood.
2. Lymph has two important functions: maintaining the body's _____ balance and providing _____ defense.
3. There are three types of lymphocytes: _____, _____, and _____.
4. The _____ immune response provides general protection to the body, and includes the skin, mucous membranes, tears, and leukocytes.

5. Lymph flows in one direction: _____ the heart.
6. The _____ is the largest lymphoid mass in the body.
7. An organ of the lymphatic system, the _____, is gradually replaced by fat and connective tissue during puberty.
8. Specific immunity can be acquired either _____ or _____.

RESPIRATORY SYSTEM

Identifying Parts of the Respiratory System
Identify the parts of the respiratory system in the image below.

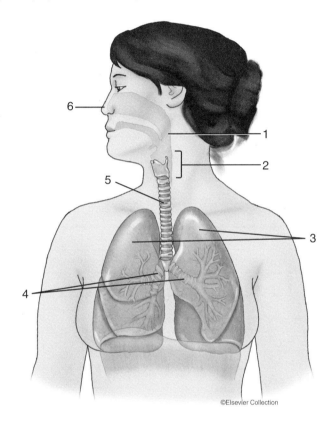

©Elsevier Collection

1. _____
2. _____
3. _____
4. _____
5. _____
6. _____

Respiratory Fill in the Blank

1. Another term for external respiration is _____.
2. Normal respiration is called _____.
3. _____ is a respiratory rate of fewer than 10 breaths per minute.
4. The _____ covers the larynx during swallowing to prevent food and/or liquid from entering the bronchi and lungs.
5. The large, flat muscle that separates the thoracic cavity from the abdominal cavity is the _____.

Chapter **6 Medical Terminology and Body Systems**

Skeletal System Fill in the Blank

Fill in each of the spaces provided with the missing word or words that complete the sentence.

1. The skeletal system consists of two major groups, called the _____ skeleton and the _____ skeleton.

2. Bones are classified by _____ as long, short, flat, or irregular.

3. The _____ cavities make the skull lighter and the voice sound stronger.

4. The _____ are openings in the cranium that close by the second year after birth.

5. Bones are joined to muscles by _____.

6. The skeletal system provides shape and support, protects internal organs, store minerals and fats, and produces _____ cells.

7. Within the bones, _____ produce new bone cells; _____ break down bone cells.

8. Most people reach peak bone density around age _____.

Classifications of Bones

Indicate the skeletal system, axial or appendicular, to which each bong belongs. Then indicate its type according to shape.

Bone	Axial or Appendicular	Long, Short, Flat, or Irregular
Lumbar vertebrae		
Ulna		
Patella		
Tarsals		
Mandible		
Scapula		
Femur		
Sternum		

Identifying the Structures of the Long Bone

Identify the structures of the long bone in the image below.

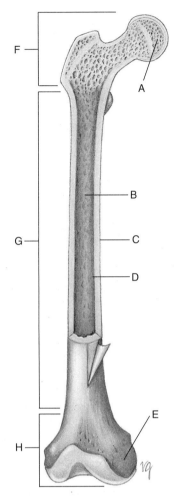

A. _____

B. _____

C. _____

D. _____

E. _____

F. _____

G. _____

H. _____

MUSCULAR SYSTEM

Muscular System Fill in the Blank

Fill in each of the spaces provided with the missing word or words that complete the sentence.

1. There are three types of muscles: skeletal, _____, and _____.

2. The _____, or agonist muscle, pulls to cause movement. Its counterpart, the _____, muscle, relaxes at the same time.

3. Skeletal muscle tissue looks striated, or _____, under the microscope.

4. Smooth muscle is controlled by the _____ nervous system.

5. _____ muscle lines various hollow organs, makes up the walls of blood vessels, and is found in the tubes of the digestive system.

6. _____ muscle is found only in the heart and is indistinctly striated.
7. Synergists and _____ are types of skeletal muscle that help stabilize bone and muscle during movement.
8. Muscles can be stimulated electrically, mechanically, or _____.
9. All types of muscle produce heat, but _____ muscle contributes most significantly to heat production in the body.
10. The walls of blood vessels are made of _____ muscle.

Identifying Muscle Tissue Type

Identify the types of muscle tissue in the images below.

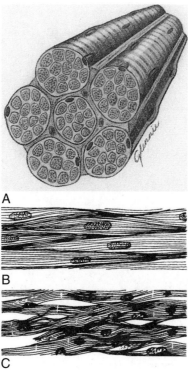

A.
B.
C.

A. _____
B. _____
C. _____

Seven Basic Types of Body Movement

Create an image of each type of movement skeletal muscles facilitate. You can use online images, cut-outs from magazines or other paper sources, or your own artistic ability. Stick figures are fine; use arrows to show the direction of movement.

DIGESTIVE SYSTEM

Digestive System Fill in the Blank

Fill in each of the spaces provided with the missing word or words that complete the sentence.
1. Another name for the digestive system is the _____ system.
2. The digestive system is not_____, as are other internal organs because it is open to the environment at both ends.
3. There are three types of salivary glands: _____; _____
   ____; and _____.

4. Another name for the throat is the _____.
5. The tube that carries food from the mouth to the stomach is the _____.
6. The three sections of the small intestine are the _____, _____ _____, and _____.
7. The large intestine has three major portions: ascending colon, _____ colon, and descending colon.
8. The different types of bacteria and microorganisms that permanently reside in our bodies and assist in our functioning are called _____.
9. _____ is composed of undigested food, mucus, bacteria, and water.

Identifying Digestive System Organs

Identify the digestive system organs in the image below.

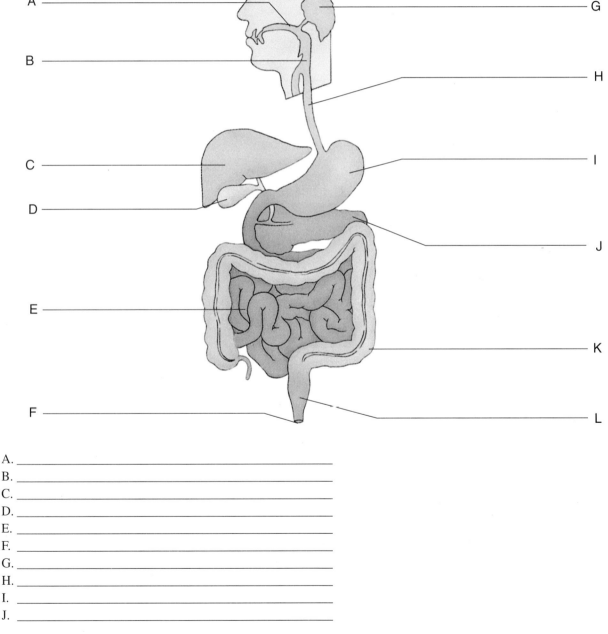

A. _____
B. _____
C. _____
D. _____
E. _____
F. _____
G. _____
H. _____
I. _____
J. _____

K. _____

L. _____

URINARY SYSTEM

Urinary System Fill in the Blank

Fill in each of the spaces provided with the missing word or words that complete the sentence.

1. Urine normally consists of _____ percent water.
2. The _____ is a tube that moves urine from the bladder to be excreted from the body via an opening called the urinary _____.
3. The _____ are small tubes that move urine from the kidney to the bladder.
4. The _____ is a smooth muscular sac that expands as it fills with urine.
5. The urinary system is also known as the _____ system.
6. The two primary functions of the urinary system are to regulate the chemical composition of body fluids and remove body wastes by filtering _____.
7. The basic structural unit of the urinary system is the _____.
8. Each kidney contains about one to two million _____, the tiny structures that filter the blood.
9. Voiding or micturition are other terms for _____.

Identifying Structures and Functions of the Urinary System

Identify the structures and functions of the urinary system in the image below.

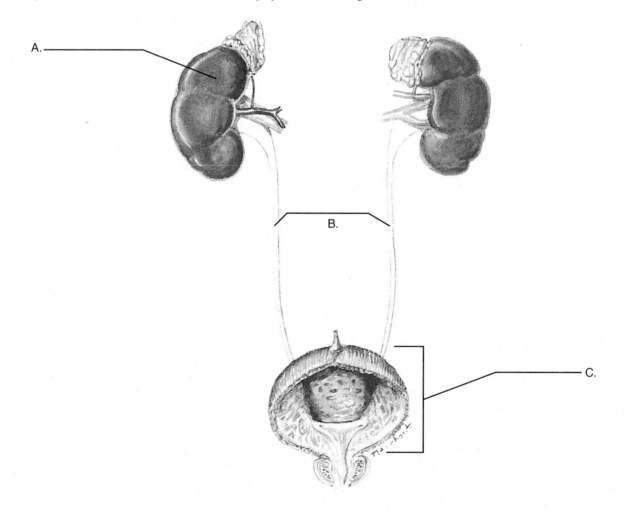

A.

B.

C.

	System Part	Main Function
A		
B		
C		

ENDOCRINE SYSTEM

Endocrine System Fill in the Blank

Fill in each of the spaces provided with the missing word or words that complete the sentence.

1. The primary function of the endocrine system is to produce _____ that monitor and coordinate body activities.
2. The _____ is a structure located above the pituitary gland that translates nervous system impulses into endocrine system messages.
3. The _____ gland has been called the "master" gland because the hormones that it produces regulate the secretion of other glands.
4. The _____ produces hormones that regulate body metabolism.
5. The _____ produces the hormones that regulate transportation of sugar, fatty acids, and amino acids into the cells.
6. When excessive secretion of growth hormone occurs in children, the resulting disorder is referred to as _____ _____.
7. The quantity of hormones in the blood is regulated through a _____ feedback mechanism.
8. The "fight-flight" reaction to stress is controlled by the _____ axis.
9. The pituitary gland is located at the base of the _____.
10. The primary sex glands, or _____, are _____ in females and _____ in males.

Endocrine Glands, Hormones, and Functions

Provide the missing information in the table.

Gland	Hormone(s)	Function
		Supports biological clock; influences secretion of sex hormones
		Increases blood calcium by releasing stored calcium in the bones
	Insulin, glucagon	
		Stimulates milk secretion and influences maternal behavior
		Maintains water balance by increasing the reabsorption of water by the kidneys

Identifying Structures of the Endocrine System

Identify the structures of the endocrine system in the image below.

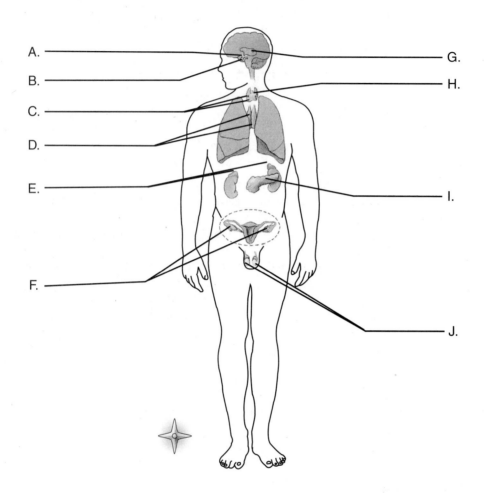

A. _____
B. _____
C. _____
D. _____
E. _____
F. _____
G. _____
H. _____
I. _____
J. _____

NERVOUS SYSTEM

Nervous System Fill in the Blank

Fill in each of the spaces provided with the missing word or words that complete the sentence.

1. The nervous system is divided into major structures: the _____ nervous system and the _____ nervous system.
2. Spinal cord nerves can act independently from the brain, as in _____ reactions, such as the knee-jerk.
3. There are _____ pairs of cranial nerves.
4. There are _____ pairs of spinal nerves.
5. The _____ nerve is a cranial nerve that also innervates various thoracic and abdominal organs.

6. Cranial nerves are divided into three groups according to the type of information carried by their fibers: sensory; _____; and _____.
7. Afferent neurons carry messages from the _____ cells of the body to the brain.
8. Efferent neurons carry messages from the _____ to the body organs or parts.
9. The autonomic nervous system is part of the _____ nervous system.
10. The dendrites, cell body, and axon are several important components of the _____.
11. The space between two neurons is called the _____.
12. The two most common _____ are acetylcholine and norepinephrine.
13. Of the four major areas of the brain, the _____ is concerned with reasoning and the senses.
14. The thalamus, the epithalamus, the subthalamus, and the hypothalamus are the four main components of the _____.
15. The _____ is sometimes referred to as the "little brain," accounting for about 10% of the total brain but containing about 50% of all the brain's neurons.
16. The structures of the _____ include the pons, medulla, and midbrain.
17. Eyes, ears, nose, tongue, and skin are all _____ organs.

Identifying Structures and Functions of the Neuron

Identify the structures and functions of the neuron in the image below.

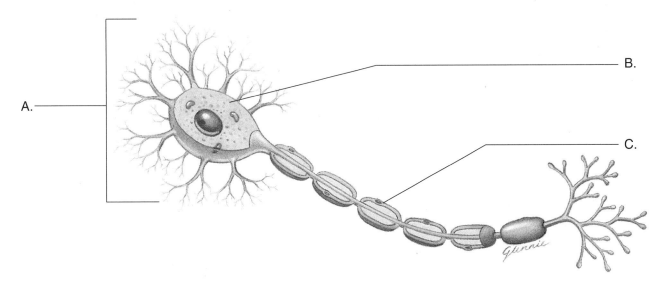

	Structure	Function(s)
A		
B		
C		

Brain Areas, Structures, and Functions

Provide the missing information in the table.

Brain Area	Brain Structure	Function(s)
	Thalamus	
Cerebrum		Personality, behavior, memory, reasoning, emotion

47

Chapter **6** **Medical Terminology and Body Systems**

Brain Area	Brain Structure	Function(s)
	Pons	
		Balance, posture, and voluntary movements; involved in muscle tone and equilibrium
	Hypothalamus	
Brainstem		Heart rate, breathing, blood pressure
		Hearing and understanding speech and printed words; memory of music and visual scenes

Sensory System Terminology

Choose the terms that match each other in meaning. Then indicate the sensory organ involved in relaying messages to the brain about these perceptions.

A	Sight
B	Hearing
C	Olfaction
D	Touch
E	Taste

1. Gustation: _____ Organ:_____
2. Tactile perception: _____ Organ:_____
3. Vision: _____ Organ:_____
4. Smell: _____ Organ:_____
5. Sound: _____ Organ:_____

REPRODUCTIVE SYSTEM

Reproductive System Fill in the Blank

Fill in each of the spaces provided with the missing word or words that complete the sentence.

1. The reproductive organs of both the male and female produce sex cells called_____.
2. _____ is the age at which the reproductive organs mature sufficiently to allow reproduction.
3. The _____ transport sperm into the ejaculatory duct below the bladder.
4. During maturation, sperm is stored in the _____.
5. From the time of conception to 2 weeks, the fertilized ovum is called a _____.
6. The process of carrying or being carried in the womb between conception and birth is called _____ _____.
7. Ovaries are glands that produce eggs as well as the two hormones, _____ and _____.
8. The _____ or inner layer of the uterus, is shed during each menstrual cycle.
9. The vagina is a muscular tube that extends from the _____ to the exterior of the body.
10. The uterus is a muscular structure in which the zygote is _____ after conception.

Identifying Structures and Functions of the Female Reproductive System

Identify the structures and functions of the female reproductive system in the image below.

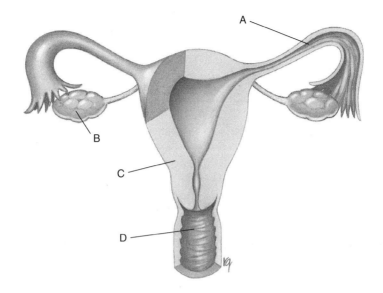

	Structure	Function(s)
A.		
B.		
C.		
D.		

Identifying Structures and Functions of the Male Reproductive System

Identify the structures and functions of the male reproductive system in the image below.

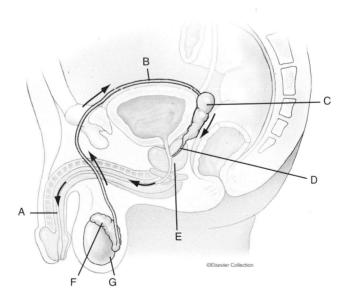

©Elsevier Collection

	Structure	Function(s)
A.		
B.		
C.		
D.		
E.		
F.		
G.		

CRITICAL THINKING

Chapter 6 has provided a wealth of information about medical terminology and body systems. What body system is most interesting to you after your reading? Why?

_____

_____

_____

_____

_____

Medical Mathematics and Calculations

KNOWLEDGE CHECK

Multiple Choice

1. Lisa misread her bill. She though it said $462.50, instead of $46.25. She likely misunderstood where the _____ was placed.
   a. denominator
   b. decimal
   c. numerator
   d. ratio

2. Total hospital admissions in 2020 were about 35 million. Of this number, 25 million were female. What is the mathematical term for representing this number as 25,000,000:10,000,000?
   a. Integer
   b. Decimal
   c. Denominator
   d. Ratio

3. For the fraction 1/5 (one-fifth, or 1 over 5), which mathematical term is the "5" called?
   a. Decimal
   b. Denominator
   c. Numerator
   d. Fraction

4. Some say the best Super Bowl in National Football League history was Super Bowl X, the Steelers versus the Cowboys. Using your knowledge of Roman numerals, what Super Bowl was this?
   a. The 1st
   b. The 5th
   c. The 10th
   d. The 50th

5. If a number needs to be rounded to the nearest hundredths, what would 0.506111 be?
   a. 0.506
   b. 0.51
   c. 0.55
   d. 0.5061

6. When multiple mathematical operations are needed for the same problem, which operation should be completed first?
   a. Anything in parentheses
   b. Any exponents
   c. Multiplication
   d. Division

7. Which is an example of a vital statistic?
   a. Ethnicities of patients seen
   b. Gender identities in a population
   c. Data about births and fetal deaths
   d. Medicare and Medicaid beneficiaries in a given population

8. Military time is based on a(n)
   a. 6-hour unit clock.
   b. 12-hour clock.
   c. 24-hour clock
   d. 8-hour clock

9. What mathematical process determines a product?
    a. Addition
    b. Multiplication
    c. Division
    d. Quotient

10. Three types of measurement systems used in healthcare are the household system, metric system, and the
    a. apothecary system.
    b. Canadian system.
    c. military system.
    d. medical system.

11. A popular acronym to remember the order of mathematical operations for a problem is
    a. "SADMEP."
    b. "PEDMAS."
    c. "PEMDAS."
    d. "MEDSAP."

12. What is 110% of 20?
    a. 55
    b. 20
    c. 25
    d. 22

13. What is 6/8 after it has been reduced?
    a. 3/8
    b. 6/4
    c. Cannot be reduced
    d. 3/4

14. A patient takes 4 pills per week. Using multiplication, how many pills will the patient take in 3 months?
    a. 24
    b. 36
    c. 42
    d. 48

15. Which profession is most likely to use the apothecary system of measurement?
    a. Nurse
    b. Contractor
    c. Pharmacist
    d. Truck driver

16. What is the answer to this problem: (5+5-1) + 8?
    a. 9
    b. 17
    c. 19
    d. 15

17. What is the answer to this problem:
    (8/2) + 116 − 20?
    a. 100
    b. 120
    c. 60
    d. 80

18. For addition, each of the numbers added together are called _____, while the end value is called the sum.
    a. values
    b. additives
    c. combiners
    d. addends

19. A number with an exponent that is positive indicates
    a. division.
    b. subtraction.
    c. addition.
    d. multiplication.

Basic Math Concepts

Match each of the following numbers to the correct meaning or answer.

Term	Meaning or Function
1. _____ 15:45	a. 13
2. _____ 4.67	b. 26
3. _____ −7	c. 0.6
4. _____ 90 mL	d. 5.25
5. _____ $(36 - 6) \div 5 + 7$	e. $5 \times 5 \times 5$
6. _____ 3/5	f. 3 oz
7. _____ $(-36 + 14)$	g. 3:45 PM
8. _____ 5^3	h. Four and sixty-seven hundredths
9. _____ 21/4	i. Seven less than zero
10. _____ XXVI	j. −22

Understanding the Concepts

1. What is the difference between a whole number and integer? Give an example of each.

_____

_____

_____

2. What are the mean, median, and mode of the following sequence of numbers?
   4, 7, 9, 3, 2, 5, 4, 9, 12, 23, 4, 6, 9, 4, 6

_____

_____

_____

_____

_____

_____

_____

_____

_____

_____

_____

_____

_____

_____

_____

MATH CALCULATIONS

Simple Operations

Compute the following problems without the use of a calculator:

1. 85,943 + 6457	2. 843 − 67	3. 345.89 + 3.02	4. 56,912 +36,891	5. 87,932 −5879	6. 834,597 −95,728
7. 367 +852 +512	8. 87 +912 +31	9. 54,873 −5825 −1804	10. 854,340 124,678 +35,956	11. 90,678 −3678 −5320	12. 76,523 78,340 + 359
13. 62 ×9	14. 403 ×34	15. 987 ×67	16. 7456 × 235	17. 47,890 × 106	18. 34,291 × 546

Division, Exponents, and Fractions

1. $265 \div 13 =$ _____

2. $56,930 \div 123 =$ _____

3. $37,893 \div 23 =$ _____

4. $78,923 \div 22 =$ _____

5. $2^3 + 3^4 =$ _____

6. $12^3 - 5^6 =$ _____

7. $6^2 \times 2^4 =$ _____

8. $7^3 \div 4^2 =$ _____

9. $36 + (5^2 - 3) =$ _____

10. $(456 - 3^3) \div 6^2 =$ _____

11. $45 - 32 + (34 \times 3) =$ _____

12. $34 \times (56 - 7^2) =$ _____

13. $^2/5 + {}^3/8 =$ _____

14. $^6/7 - {}^2/9 =$ _____

15. $^5/6 \times {}^3/4 =$ _____

16. $^7/8 \div {}^2/3 =$ _____

USING MATH IN HEALTHCARE

Converting Temperature

Convert the temperature measurements.

1. $35°C =$ _____ $°F$

2. $98.4°F =$ _____ $°C$

3. $33.5°C =$ _____ $°F$

4. $100.2°F =$ _____ $°C$

Word Problems

1. How many cups of water should your patient drink in 8 hours if the doctor has ordered 1000 cc?

_____

_____

2. How much does a patient weigh in pounds if the scale reads 65 kg?

_____

_____

3. For breakfast your patient consumes a cup of gelatin, 1/2 cup of coffee, 2/3 glass of juice, and 1/2 cup of ice cubes. What intake should you record for this meal?

_____

_____

4. The doctor has instructed your patient to wear an eye patch at least 10 hours daily while awake. The patient sleeps 7 hours each night and does not want to wear the eye patch to school (8:00 AM to 3:00 PM). With these limitations, can the patient wear the eye patch for 10 hours?

_____

_____

5. If you spend 30 minutes to give morning care (bath and bed change) for each patient, how long with it take you to give care to 8 patients?

_____

_____

6. The CDC recommends using a 1:10 (household bleach to water) solution to disinfect hard surfaces such as floors. How much bleach should you add to a gallon of water to make this solution?

_____

_____

STATISTICS IN HEALTH CARE

Health Care Statistics

Rates are an expression of how often something occurs. The calculation for any rate is a simple one: how often something happened (for a given period of time) divided by the number of times it could have happened (in that same time period). The numerator is the times the event occurred, and the denominator is the number of times it could have occurred. The result is multiplied by 100 to express the rate as a percentage. Using the formulas in Box 7-1, read the scenario and answer the questions that follow.

Box 7-1 Rate Formulas for Selected Institutional Statistics

$$\frac{count\ of\ the\ event\ for\ a\ time\ period}{Number\ of\ times\ it\ could\ have\ occured\ in\ the\ time\ period} \times 100 = Rate$$

Calculating a Healthcare-Associated Infection Rate

$$\frac{Total\ number\ of\ infections\ after\ 48\ hours\ of\ hospitalization\ for\ a\ period}{Total\ number\ of\ discharges\ (including\ deaths)\ for\ a\ period} \times 100$$

Calculating Caesarean-section Rates

$$\frac{(Total\ number\ of\ Caeserean\ sections\ for\ a\ period)}{(Total\ number\ of\ deliveries\ (live\ or\ dead)\ for\ this\ period)} \times 100$$

Calculating Newborn Mortality Rates

$$\frac{Total\ number\ of\ newborn\ deaths\ for\ a\ period}{Total\ number\ of\ newborn\ discharges\ (including\ deaths)\ for\ this\ period} \times 100$$

At the community hospital, 919 women delivered 943 babies. Five infants died postpartum in the newborn period. Twenty-four babies were multiples. Obstetricians performed 291 Caesarean section, or C-sections. Two women developed infections after their C-sections.

1. What is the C-section rate as a percentage rounded to the nearest 100th?
2. What is the newborn mortality rate as a percentage rounded to the nearest 100th?
3. What is the healthcare associate infection rate for C-sections as a percentage rounded to the nearest 100th?

8 Health Insurance and the Revenue Cycle

Multiple Choice

1. At what point does the revenue cycle begin?
   a. When services are rendered
   b. When the insurer receives claim
   c. When the patient makes an appointment
   d. When the patient receives a bill

2. Dr Smith's office formally requested payment from his patient's insurance company for services he provided. This is called a
   a. premium.
   b. preauthorization.
   c. claim.
   d. formulary.

3. Blue Cross Blue Shield, Aetna, Medicaid and Medicare are examples of
   a. first-party payers.
   b. second-party payers.
   c. third-party payers.
   d. tertiary payers.

4. Three weeks after he had an MRI, Mr Lewis received a statement showing an amount that was not covered by insurance. What is this statement?
   a. Formulary
   b. Explanation of benefits
   c. Beneficiary description statement
   d. Subscriber report

5. A *subscriber* is someone who purchases and is covered by private insurance. What is the term for a person covered by a government payer?
   a. Group insured person
   b. Second-party payee
   c. Claimant
   d. Beneficiary

6. The Davidsons have private insurance coverage for their whole family. They pay a(n) _____ of $400 per month to keep the coverage active.
   a. copay
   b. premium
   c. deductible
   d. indemnity

7. The Davidsons also have to pay $2000 worth of services out-of-pocket each year, before insurance will "kick in" and start covering future medical costs. This $2000 is called a(n)
   a. annuity.
   b. deductible.
   c. copayment or copay.
   d. coinsurance.

8. Typically, insurance plans with higher deductibles will have lower
   a. premiums.
   b. coverage.
   c. out-of-pocket costs.
   d. lifetime maximums.

57

9. Rita has been prescribed a new medication. She should check her insurance company's _____ to make sure the drug is covered under her plan.
   a. explanation of benefits
   b. managed care policy
   c. formulary
   d. ICD-10 statement

10. What is the term for the type of insurance that is known as fee-for-service or conventional insurance?
    a. Cost-sharing
    b. Managed care
    c. Indemnity
    d. Health Maintenance Organization (HMO)

11. What is the name of the legislation that is considered of the most significant healthcare reforms since Medicare and Medicaid?
    a. Alternative Care Act (ACA)
    b. Alternative Compensation Act (ACA)
    c. American Care Act (ACA)
    d. Affordable Care Act (ACA)

12. *Managed care* was introduced in the 1970s to cut costs by
    a. limiting the providers the patient can see.
    b. covering fewer sick people, as they are more expensive to provide coverage for.
    c. offering fewer covered services.
    d. only covering elective procedures.

13. In what year were Medicare and Medicaid enacted in the United States?
    a. 1935
    b. 2020
    c. 1965
    d. 2000

14. The Centers for Medicare and Medicaid Services enforces a cap called a *limiting charge*. This rule states that a provider cannot charge more than _____ of Medicare's approved amount.
    a. 100%
    b. 115%
    c. 125%
    d. 120%

15. What is "Medigap"?
    a. The difference between Medicare and Medicaid
    b. A supplemental insurance policy that covers things that standard Medicare will not cover
    c. The range of ages for people who qualify for Medicare services
    d. The difference between what providers charge private insurance subscribers and Medicare beneficiaries

16. Medicaid is health coverage for whom?
    a. People in poverty
    b. Veterans
    c. People injured at work
    d. Orphans

17. Medical coding, or coding for short, translates diagnoses and treatments into
    a. short statements.
    b. abbreviated terms.
    c. readable text.
    d. strings of alphanumeric and numeric characters.

18. The ICD-10-CM coding system is used by providers, research organizations, billers, and coders in over 100 countries and features 68,000 codes. They are used to represent
    a. procedures.
    b. services provided.
    c. medical products (DMEs).
    d. diagnoses.

19. The coding system that translates medical products, supplies, and services into codes is
    a. ICD-10-CM.
    b. ICD-10-PCS.

    c. HCPCS.

    d. ICD-10-DME.

20. What are *Evaluation and management (E/M) codes* used for?

    a. To standardize administrative employee actions and services

    b. To represent various levels of physician service provided

    c. As an alternative to ICD-10-CM codes

    d. To represent the performance of the management of a clinic

True/False

Read the following statements and write "T" for true or "F" for false in the blanks provided. If a statement is false, correct the statement to make it true.

_____ 1. Precertification, preauthorization, and predetermination are all terms that refer to the process of obtaining approval from the insurer for a service before the service is performed.

_____ 2. Typically, a copay is the same amount, whether the patient sees a doctor for a wellness exam or goes to the emergency department for a broken leg.

_____ 3. The revenue cycle is a set of investment decisions associated with increasing income for managed care organizations.

_____ 4. Indemnity insurance is also referred to as "fee-for-service" insurance.

_____ 5. If a patient has a deductible of $2500, they must spend $2000 out-of-pocket, starting at the beginning of the year, before their insurance will start covering medical bills.

_____ 6. Managed care insurers steer their large pool of patients to specific providers, which gives the providers a stable group of patients.

_____ 7. Medicare is offered to people 65 years and older, as well as people with certain disabilities.

_____ 8. Many insurance companies follow TRICARE guidelines when adopting reimbursement strategies.

_____ 9. Evaluation and management (E/M) codes are divided into two levels: routine and complex.

_____ 10. As of 2020, ICD-10 is the current edition of the International Classification of Diseases. The next revision will be ICD-11.

REVENUE CYCLE

Revenue Cycle Visualization

Using the textbook and other sources, create a visual representation, such as a diagram or flowchart, of the revenue cycle for a healthcare facility or provider's office. You can use any medium you like (i.e., digital or paper). For each step, include the individuals who participate in it and their roles.

HEALTH INSURANCE

Fill in the Blank

Fill in each of the spaces provided with the missing word or words that complete the sentence.

1. The first medical insurance company in the United States was _____.

2. Deductibles, copayments, and coinsurance are all forms of _____ of insurance.

3. Seeing a(n) _____ provider, as opposed to one outside the insurance plan's group of providers, typically means the patient will pay a lower copayment.

4. Many insurances have a(n) _____ limit that is the maximum amount patients must pay for their own healthcare annually.

5. The Affordable Care Act removed lifetime maximums for _____ benefits.

6. Member, enrollee, and covered life are terms used for a patient who is part of a _____ organization.

7. The MCO doesn't dictate what care is provided; it dictates what care it will _____.

8. In a(n) _____ HMO, individual physicians contract with the HMO and devote part of their practices to seeing HMO enrollees.

9. In the year _____, President Obama signed the Patient Protection and Affordable Care Act into law.

10. In 2017, the U.S. Supreme Court eliminated the _____ of the Affordable Care Act, so that Americans were no longer forced to purchase health insurance.

Pricing Health Insurance

Research health insurance prices in your area. Healthcare.gov is a good website to use, or check with other health insurance companies. Compare three plans based on premium, deductible, copayments, and coverage.

Plan 1	Premium	
	Deductible	
	Copayments	
	Coverage	
Plan 2	Premium	
	Deductible	
	Copayments	
	Coverage	
Plan 3	Premium	
	Deductible	
	Copayments	
	Coverage	

GOVERNMENT HEALTHCARE COVERAGE

Programs and Administrators

Using the textbook and other sources, fill in the missing information in the table of federal healthcare programs.

Program	Description	Coverage	Administrator
	Medical services for active-duty members of the armed services, their spouses and families, and retirees under the age of 65	Members of Army, Air Force, Navy, Marine Corps, Coast Guard, Public Health Service, and the National Oceanic and Atmospheric Administration Force, Navy, Marine Corps, Coast Guard, Public Health Service, and the National Oceanic and Atmospheric Administration	
CHIP			Administered by states according to federal regulations
	Civilian Health and Medical Program of the Department of Veterans Affairs		
IHS			
Medicaid	Title XIX of the Social Security Act of 1965	Low-income families and the medically needy	
Medicare			Centers for Medicare and Medicaid Services
VHA		U.S. veterans	

Medicare, Medicaid, and the Affordable Care Act

Healthcare policy and reform are not new topics in the United States. Although the Affordable Care Act was passed in 2010, two other forms of government-sponsored healthcare insurance were established in 1965: Medicare and Medicaid. Read more about these programs, and then, using those sources and other government websites, answer these questions.

Links:

Medicare history: https://www.ssa.gov/history/ssa/lbjmedicare1.html

Medicaid history: https://www.medicaid.gov/about-us/program-history/index.html

Read the following statements and write "T" for true or "F" for false in the blanks provided. If a statement is false, correct the statement to make it true.

1. ____ Prior to the establishment of Medicare, only older people with substantial incomes and savings were truly safe from the prospect of financial disaster posed by a severe illness.
2. ____ Medicare was initially comprised of two related health insurance plans for persons aged 65 or older.
3. ____ It took 8 years between enactment of the Social Security Amendment of 1965 and the start of its operations.
4. ____ President John F. Kennedy signed the Medicare legislation into law.
5. ____ As with Medicare, the federal government administers the Medicaid program.
6. ____ The Children's Health Insurance Program provides health coverage to children in families with incomes too high to qualify for Medicaid, but unable to afford private health insurance.
7. ____ The Affordable Care Act allows states to expand Medicaid eligibility to people under age 65 in families with incomes below 200% of the Federal Poverty Line.
8. ____ The original premium for Medicare was $3 a month.

Understanding the Federal Poverty Line

Using a government website, find the current Federal Poverty Line (FPL) for a family of 4 and record it here:

48 States and District of Columbia:_____

Alaska:_____

Hawaii:_____

State of your choice: _____

Was the FPL in line with what you expected? Why or why not?

_____

_____

_____

_____

_____

HEALTHCARE CLASSIFICATION SYSTEMS AND CODE SETS

Match each characteristic, service, procedure, or diagnosis with the classification system or code set to which it belongs. Answers may be used more than once.

ICD-10-CM
ICD-10-PCS
CPT
HCPCS Level II
E/M Codes

1. Approximately 68,000 codes   _____
2. Ambulance interventions   _____
3. Chest pain   _____
4. X-ray in doctor's office   _____

5. Partial nephrectomy (kidney removal) _____
6. Problem-focused exam _____
7. Decimal point after first three figures _____
8. Used only in inpatient and hospital settings _____
9. Complete examination of single organ system _____
10. Medications _____

CRITICAL THINKING

Healthcare: A Right or a Privilege?

Access to healthcare is a hotly debated topic. Politicians, religious leaders, human rights activists, and ethicists (not to mention friends, relatives, and family members) all have something to say about the concept of healthcare as either a right or a privilege. Some argue that healthcare is a basic human right, one that should be provided for every individual regardless of income, race, gender, ethnicity, or any other factor. Others counter that healthcare is a privilege that, like other commodities, is available to those who can afford it, and that no individual is responsible for the healthcare consumption decisions or needs of others.

1. In general, do you think healthcare is a right or a privilege? Why?

_____
_____
_____
_____
_____
_____
_____
_____
_____

2. Do you think personal behaviors such as tobacco and alcohol use, lack of exercise, or riding a bike without a helmet should influence how much an individual pays for health insurance? Why or why not?

_____
_____
_____
_____
_____
_____
_____
_____
_____
_____

9 Healthcare Technology and EHR

KNOWLEDGE CHECK

Multiple Choice

1. In addition to medical and clinical documentation, a patient's medical record includes
   a. federal and state tax information.
   b. the patient's wages from work.
   c. the patient's demographic information.
   d. the patient's DNA profile.

2. Within a clinic, the core purpose of the patient's medical record is
   a. organization.
   b. communication.
   c. transferal.
   d. referral.

3. What is the term for the quality of the provision of health care given to a person over time, sometimes from multiple providers?
   a. Sustained services
   b. Constant care
   c. Continuity of care
   d. Consistency of care

4. The EHR makes data collection easier through
   a. open access to any individual.
   b. robust reporting functions.
   c. dropdown menus and radio buttons.
   d. data sharing with the Nationwide Health Information Network (NHIN).

5. Which of these is only possible in the EHR, not in a paper medical record?
   a. Correcting the record
   b. Adding notes of the record
   c. Allowing two providers in different locations to view the record simultaneously
   d. Reviewing a patient's record for billing purposes

6. What is the name of the feature of an EHR record that lets providers select and officially request lab work, images, and prescriptions?
   a. Communication-adapted pharmacy order entry (CPOE)
   b. Computer-assisted physician order entry (CPOE)
   c. Computer-assisted provider obedience engine (CPOE)
   d. Completion-able provider order entry (CPOE)

7. What will the EHR software do if a provider's selected order triggers a contraindication?
   a. The system will shut down.
   b. The system will choose something else.
   c. The system will alert the provider.
   d. The system will inform the patient directly.

8. Clinical protocols are _____ plans of care for patients with specific problems.
   a. experimental
   b. preventative
   c. simple
   d. standardized

9. Which component of the EHR recommends treatment protocols to providers?
   a. Electronic document management system (EDMS)
   b. Clinical decision support system (CDS)
   c. Computer-assisted physician order entry (CPOE)
   d. Practice management software (PMS)

63

10. Which term means the tracking and tracing of everyone who has accessed a patient's electronic health record?
    a. Health portability
    b. Remote fingerprinting
    c. Contraindication protocol
    d. Audit trail

11. Which term refers to the part of an EHR that allows patients to log into their medical record and view certain information or message their provider?
    a. Provider portal
    b. Patient portal
    c. Patient coding
    d. Provider coding

12. Coding documents diagnoses, procedures, and other services using
    a. abbreviations.
    b. numeric and alphanumeric characters.
    c. Latin words.
    d. short-hand medical terms

13. In order for health care facilities' EHR software to work together, they must be
    a. longitudinal.
    b. accurate.
    c. private.
    d. interoperable.

14. Interoperability between the EHRs of varied organizations is referred to as a(n)
    a. administrative network.
    b. health information exchange.
    c. compatibility communication connection.
    d. remote patient mainframe.

15. A _____ allows the provider to search the database of another provider and access patient information.
    a. directed exchange
    b. consumer-mediated exchange
    c. query-based exchange
    d. patient portal

16. Which type of health information exchange (HIE) lets patients send their information to other networked providers?
    a. Query-based exchange
    b. Consumer-mediated exchange
    c. Directed exchange
    d. Private patient exchange

17. The Office of the National Coordinator for Health Information Technology (ONC) promotes, at a federal level, the
    a. increased adoption of EHR software and interoperability.
    b. decreased need for EHR software.
    c. the decrease in cost of EHRs.
    d. number of patients seen in rural areas.

18. Telehealth via live video makes the _____ of the patient irrelevant.
    a. health
    b. ability to pay
    c. language
    d. location

19. Which form of telehealth involves a provider reviewing pre-recorded video or images at a later time?
    a. Multimedia
    b. Virtual appointment
    c. Store-and-forward
    d. Real-time audiovisual

20. Mrs Bailey is a diabetic who uses remote patient monitoring (RPM) to
   a. transmit her blood glucose level to her doctor.
   b. have video appointments with her provider.
   c. keep her own records of insulin injections.
   d. adjust her medications.

True/False

Read the following statements and write "T" for true or "F" for false in the blanks provided. If a statement is false, correct the statement to make it true.

1. ____ Data from the EHR regarding clinical quality measures is reported to the Office of the National Coordinator for Health Information Technology (ONC), which uses it to inform policy decisions.

2. ____ A prescription from a doctor's official prescription pad is likely safer and more accurate than if it was sent by CPOE.

3. ____ EHRs improve quality of care by ensuring the providers complete audit trails, such as screening for depression.

4. ____ Patient management software can easily generate personalized legal forms.

5. ____ The benefit of a longitudinal health record is that it lets healthcare professionals see the big picture, or whole story, of a patient.

6. ____ Billing and patient management systems that are incorporated into EHR can complete medical billing, eliminating the need for medical billing and coding professionals.

7. ____ Most healthcare providers that have a business relationship use the directed exchange form of health information exchange.

8. ____ The non-profit Sequoia Project manages the nation's largest health information exchange, which connects about 10% of U.S. hospitals.

9. ____ Health Level 7 has been creating and selling EHR software since its founding in 1987.

10. ____ Telehealth has been around for decades.

THE ELECTRONIC HEALTH RECORD

Features and Benefits of EHR Technology

Using the textbook and other sources, answer each of the questions in your own words.

1. The format used in EHRs depends on the setting, specialty, patient population, and sometimes the preference of the healthcare provider. Give an example of how one or more of these factors might influence the format of the EHR.

_____

_____

_____

_____

_____

_____

2. What is the purpose of an audit trail in an EHR system?

_____

_____

_____

_____

_____

_____

3. What are some of the basic ways the use of an EHR system reduces medical errors?

_____

_____

_____

_____

_____

_____

Administrative Functions

Using the textbook and other sources, answer each of the questions in your own words.

1. What information is collected and input into patient management software during patient registration?

_____

_____

_____

_____

2. Patient management software uses a calendar interface to schedule appointments. How does the software remind patients of their appointments?

_____

_____

_____

_____

3. After a claim has been sent electronically to the third-party payer or insurer, what role does billing software have in the revenue cycle?

_____

_____

_____

_____

HEALTH INFORMATION EXCHANGES

Benefits of HIEs

Using the textbook and other sources, review the advantages of the health information exchange. List them here.

_____

_____

_____

_____

_____

_____

Sequoia Project

The non-profit Sequoia Project engages with government and industry to identify and remove barriers to interoperability. Its initiatives include PULSE (Patient Unified Lookup System for Emergencies), RSNA Image Share Validation, Carequality, and eHealth Exchange. Using the link in the textbook, research one of these initiatives and answer the following questions.

1. Which initiative did you choose?

   _____

2. What is the purpose of the initiative?

   _____

   _____

   _____

   _____

   _____

3. What is an example of the initiative in action? (This information might be obtained through links to news articles, featured users, or testimonials on the initiative's website.)

   _____

   _____

   _____

   _____

   _____

   _____

TELEHEALTH

Benefits of Telehealth

Using the textbook and other sources, list three patient populations that might benefit from telehealth services, and explain why?

1. _____

   _____

   _____

   _____

2. _____

   _____

   _____

   _____

3. _____

_____

_____

_____

CRITICAL THINKING

Should Insurers Pay for Telehealth?

1. Before the COVID-19 pandemic, Medicare would not reimburse providers for services delivered via telehealth. In the interest of social distancing and reducing the transmission of the virus, Centers for Medicare and Medicaid Services (CMS) added telehealth coverage for certain services, and some private insurers have done the same. Why do you think Medicare has been reluctant to cover telehealth expenses except under these specific circumstances?

_____

_____

_____

_____

_____

_____

_____

_____

_____

2. In general, do you think third-party payers, including Medicare, should reimburse providers for telehealth? Why or why not?

_____

_____

_____

_____

_____

_____

_____

_____

_____

_____

10 Basic Accounting and Finance

KNOWLEDGE CHECK

Multiple Choice

Circle the one correct answer to each of the following questions.

1. The medical office manager is reviewing the organization's bank statement online and the debit column contains subtractions of funds from the account. What is the name of the column where money is added?
   a. Accounts payable (A/P)
   b. Accounts receivable (A/R)
   c. Credit
   d. Asset

2. The amount of money held in a bank account, which you are technically letting the bank borrow from you, is referred to as the _____, and interest can be paid to you based on this amount.
   a. statement
   b. principal
   c. posting
   d. budget

3. A money market account is meant to
   a. hold a small amount of money accessed frequently.
   b. hold a large amount of money accessed infrequently.
   c. house tax-free contributions that may not be withdrawn until the account holder turns 59½.
   d. be used to purchase stocks, bonds, and other investments.

4. Paychecks are most often distributed via automated clearing house (ACH) transfers, also known as
   a. instant checks.
   b. direct distributions.
   c. direct deposits.
   d. electronic deposits.

5. Mr Ripley has $550 in his checking account and wrote a check for $750; he will likely incur a(n) _____ penalty.
   a. subzero
   b. indebtedness
   c. overdraft
   d. underbalance

6. What is the name for the process of ensuring that your record of transactions matches the bank's records?
   a. Posting
   b. Revenue streaming
   c. Expensing
   d. Reconciliation

7. Which financial statement is a record of all the monies charged and collected that day?
   a. Balance sheet
   b. Checking register
   c. Day sheet
   d. Patient ledger

8. Which accounting method reports transactions when money physically moves, not when services are rendered?
   a. Accrual basis accounting
   b. Cash basis accounting
   c. Fiscal accounting
   d. Balance sheet accounting

9. The United Way is a not-for-profit organization that pools fundraising efforts for various charities. If they have income that is above their expenses, it is called
   a. net profit.

69

    b. net income.

    c. gross profit.

    d. residual income.

10. When the fiscal year aligns with the calendar year, the 4th quarter is from

    a. October 1st to December 31st.

    b. November 1st to December 31st.

    c. September 1st to December 31st.

    d. November 1st to January 1st of the following year.

11. Where are employee salaries listed on a balance sheet?

    a. Debits

    b. Assets

    c. Liabilities

    d. Accounts receivable (A/R)

12. Which is the correct equation used to ensure assets, liabilities, and net worth equal out on a balance sheet?

    a. Assets = Liabilities + Net Worth

    b. Assets = Net worth – Liabilities

    c. Assets = Accounts Payable + Salary

    d. Assets = Liabilities – Net Worth

13. Which of these items owned by Hempstead Community Hospital is a fixed asset?

    a. Inventory

    b. Cash

    c. Accounts receivable

    d. Hospital beds

14. The change in the value of fixed assets over time is called

    a. inflation.

    b. deflation.

    c. depreciation.

    d. demarcation.

15. Kesher Hospital spent $800,000 on a state-of-the art MRI machine capable of generating functional MRI images (fMRIs). They expect to have this fixed asset for 10 years. Due to depreciation, how much will this machine's net value be in the second year?

    a. $700,000

    b. $400,000

    c. $720,000

    d. $790,000

16. What is another term for an income statement?

    a. Positive and negative statement

    b. Profit and loss statement

    c. Asset and liability statement

    d. Accounts receivable statement

17. In a healthcare facility, which component typically represents the largest portion of accounts receivable (A/R)?

    a. Vendor accounts

    b. Patient accounts

    c. Inventory

    d. Medicaid revenue

18. What is the correct formula for calculating net worth?

    a. Net Worth = Assets – Liabilities

    b. Net Worth = Cash + Debts

    c. Net Worth = Liabilities + Assets

    d. Net Worth = Accounts Receivable (A/R) – Account Payable (A/P)

19. In regard to budgeting, what is the term for a large, one-time purchase?

    a. Sole expenditure or "sopex"

    b. Capital expenditure or "capex"

    c. Major expenditure or "maxex"

    d. Chief expenditure or "chex"

20. What is the term for how long an equipment purchase will take to pay itself off?

    a. Lease time

b. Retribution period
c. Interest recovery period
d. Payback period

21. In contrast to the capital expenditure budget, what is the name for the amount designated for payroll, utility bills, and office supplies?
a. Daily budget
b. Fiscal budget
c. Annual budget
d. Operational budget

22. What is the term for expenses that can be counted on to stay the same month-to-month?
a. Variable costs
b. Fixed costs
c. Annual costs
d. Flexible costs

23. Sick pay and retirement contributions are called
a. French benefits.
b. edge benefits.
c. fringe benefits.
d. bridge benefits.

24. Harrison Hospital budgeted $500,000 for its innovations department but actually spent $550,000. What is this difference called?
a. Variance
b. Split
c. Separation
d. Influx

25. Income statements include all the ways a company generates money, called
a. revenue paths.
b. payment paths.
c. revenue streams.
d. income surges.

True/False

Read the following statements and write "T" for true or "F" for false in the blanks provided. If a statement is false, correct the statement to make it true.

_____ 1. Credit card companies only make money if the consumers who use them do not pay off their balances in full each month.

_____ 2. Although there are no laws regarding the maintenance of financial records, it is imperative that a business records transactions to understand its successes and failures.

_____ 3. Reconciliation of a bank statement includes totaling any outstanding deposits or checks on record at the facility that have not yet been processed at the bank.

_____ 4. The terms "revenue" and "profit" are synonymous.

_____ 5. For-profit and not-for-profit are terms that refer to the tax status of an organization.

_____ 6. A patient ledger, or patient account, keeps track of what an individual patient was charged, how much the patient has paid, and how much the patient still owes.

_____ 7. In accounting terms, a credit is when you charge an amount and pay it off at a later date.

_____ 8. The matching principle is used with cash basis accounting.

_____ 9. Monitoring accounts receivable is a way for a facility to track money that has been counted as revenue, but that has not actually been received yet.

_____ 10. The aging report is a subset of accounts payable that are overdue.

_____ 11. Most companies typically divide their fiscal year into quarters.

_____ 12. Net income means the amount before any deductions are made.

_____ 13. If an asset is deemed "current," that means it has to be used within one year.

_____ 14. Prepaid expenses are usually paid for in six-month increments.

_____ 15. The portion of a long-term debt that is due within the coming year is considered a long-term liability.

_____ 16. Accountants for healthcare businesses choose one of two types of budgets: capital or operational.

_____ 17. An expense that is accounted for in an operational budget is equipment leasing costs.

_____ 18. Variances are usually reported on a monthly basis.

71

Interest-Bearing Accounts

This chapter discussed three types of interest-bearing accounts: savings, checking, and money market. Research the interest rates on these types of accounts at two financial institutions. Bankrate.com, MagnifyMoney.com, and NerdWallet.com are some websites that provide comparisons among institutions. What, if any, requirements must be met to earn the interest rates for the three types of accounts at each institution? Do the institutions charge any fees associated with the accounts? Record your findings.

		Financial Institution #1 Name	Financial Institution #2 Name
Interest Rate	SVG		
	CKG		
	MM		
Requirements	SVG		
	CKG		
	MM		
Fees	SVG		
	CKG		
	MM		

SVG = Savings, CKG = Checking, MM = Money Market.

Parts of a Check

Paper checks are not as common as they once were, but you will encounter them when working in the business office of a healthcare facility. Name each numbered part of the check shown.

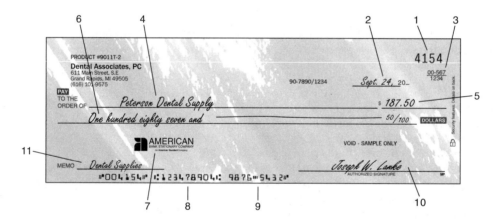

1. _____
2. _____
3. _____
4. _____
5. _____
6. _____
7. _____
8. _____

9. _____

10. _____

11. _____

Reconciling a Bank Statement

Using the worksheet below and the bank statement in Figure 10-1, follow the steps below to reconcile the bank statement.

Ms Stankowski's checkbook balance is $4,019.01, not the closing amount shown on the bank statement. She has one outstanding deposit for $250.00, and she has written checks for $1000.00, $200.00, $100.00, and $227.76 that have not cleared.

1. List ending the closing balance on the bank statement balance		$ _____
2. Subtract outstanding checks (written but not cleared)	-	$ _____
3. Add deposits not shown on statement	+	$ _____
4. TOTAL (corrected bank statement balance)	=	$ _____
5. List corrected checkbook balance (should match amount in Step 4)		$ ____$3,999.01_____
6. Subtract any bank charges/fees	-	$ _____
7. Corrected checkbook balance	=	$ _____

Your Favorite Bank
1234 Main St.
Anytown, XY 12345

Sheila Stankowski
878 Oak St.
Anytown, XY 12345

Account Number: 123-4257896
Period Covered: 03/15/20XX to 04/18/20XX

Account Summary

Opening Balance	$4,275.90
Withdrawals	$2,345.00
Deposits	$3,345.87

Closing Balance on April 18, 20XX   **$5,276.77**

Transaction Details

Date	Description	Withdrawals	Deposits	Balance
04/01/20XX	Opening Balance			4275.90
04/04/20XX	Direct Debit Venmo Payment	300.00		3975.90
04/04/20XX	Direct Deposit		3245.87	7721.77
04/06/20XX	Check Paid # 1458 (Cash)	1160.50		6061.27
04/08/20XX	Check Paid # 1460 (Cash)	20.00		6041.27
04/11/20XX	Returned Check Fee	20.00		6021.27
04/12/20XX	Check Paid # 1457 (Cash)	100.00		5921.27
04/12/20XX	Direct Debit CGI Utility AUTOPAY	236.65		5684.62
04/15/20XX	Deposit		100.00	5784.62
04/16/20XX	Direct Debit Credit Card AUTOPAY	507.85		5276.77
	Closing Balance			**$5,276.77**

Figure 10-1 Sample Bank Statement.

Chapter **10 Basic Accounting and Finance**

BOOKKEEPING AND ACCOUNTING

Bookkeeping vs Accounting

Many people working in healthcare administration are trained in accounting and finance. Research bookkeeping and accounting, and then answer these questions. The Bureau of Labor Statistics (www.bls.gov) maintains an online Occupational Outlook Handbook that is a good source of information.

1. What are the basic responsibilities of a bookkeeper?

_____

_____

_____

2. What are the basic responsibilities of an accountant?

_____

_____

_____

3. What education and training is necessary to become a bookkeeper?

_____

_____

_____

4. What education and training is necessary to become an accountant?

_____

_____

_____

5. What is the compensation range for a bookkeeper in your area?

_____

6. What is the compensation range for an accountant in your area?

_____

Electronic Health Records and Billing

Many healthcare providers use electronic health record (EHR) software that features built-in accounting capabilities. Smaller medical practices—may not have an integrated EHR and billing system, but nearly all will use special accounting software.

Research software that integrates accounting with EHR. Many companies' websites provide a brief demo video that may be helpful.

1. What company did you research? _____

2. How did you find it? _____

3. What were some of the features of the software you liked?

_____

_____

_____

4. What size provider do you think this software would be good for? Why?

_____

_____

_____

Cash Basis vs Accrual Basis Accounting

The textbook described two basic methods of accounting: cash basis and accrual basis. Cash basis accounting reports transactions when the money physically moves. It records income when the patient's bill is paid, not when the service is rendered. Accrual basis accounting reports transactions at the time the services are performed. In a medical setting that uses accrual basis accounting, income is reported when the patient is seen and services are rendered, regardless of when the patient pays the bill.

What are two advantages of each method of accounting?

Cash Basis

1. _____
2. _____

Accrual Basis

1. _____
2. _____

FINANCIAL REPORTS

Fiscal Year

List three reasons a company might choose a fiscal year calendar that differs from the regular calendar year.

1. _____
2. _____
3. _____

Balance Sheet

A balance sheet shows how much an organization is worth. It includes the assets of a company, the liabilities associated with those assets and the general business operation, and the company's net worth. As a reminder, net worth is the difference between your assets and your liabilities (Net Worth = Assets – Liabilities).

Individuals and families also create balance sheets to understand their financial position. Create your own personal balance sheet. You can use Figure 10-2, or a spreadsheet program such as Excel. Do not be concerned about calculating depreciation of your assets but do consider whether they are current or fixed. Similarly, decide whether your liabilities are short or long term.

This document will be for your own reference; you will not share it with the instructor or your classmates.

Questions

1. If your total worth is more than your total debt, what would be a good way to invest the excess income?

_____

_____

_____

2. If your total worth is less than your total debt, what would be a source of additional money or an expense that could be cut?

_____

_____

_____

BUDGETING

Personal Budget

Using the information gained from creating your balance sheet, create a personal budget for a period of time. Typically, budgets are monthly, but you can work with a shorter or longer time period if you'd prefer. You can use Figure 10-3 to record your budget, or there are a number of good budgeting apps available, as well as online guides and books.

This document will be for your own reference; you will not share it with the instructor or your classmates.

PERSONAL FINANCIAL STATEMENT

Owned:

Cash	$ _____
Securities (stocks, bonds, CDs)	$ _____ *
Real estate	$ _____ *
Automobile	$ _____ *
Furniture	$ _____ *
Receivables (money owed to you)	$ _____
Other	$ _____

Total Owned: $ _____

Owed:

Household bills unpaid	$ _____
Installment payments:	
Automobile	$ _____
Appliances	$ _____
Loans	$ _____
Other	$ _____
Real estate payments	$ _____
Insurance:	
Automobile	$ _____
Personal property	$ _____
Health	$ _____
Other	$ _____
Taxes	$ _____
Other debts	$ _____

Total Owed: $ _____

Total Owned Minus Total Owed Equals Total Worth = $ _____

*Value should be determined by the amount that could be obtained from a quick sale.

Figure 10-2

Regular or Fixed Monthly Payments*

Mortgage or rent	$ _____
Automobile payment	$ _____
Automobile insurance	$ _____
Appliance	$ _____
Loan	$ _____
Health insurance	$ _____
Personal property insurance	$ _____
Telephone	$ _____
Utilities (gas or electric)	$ _____
Water	$ _____
Other non-emergency expenses	$ _____

Discretionary or Variable Payments

Clothing, laundry, cleaning	$ _____
Medicine	$ _____
Doctor and dentist	$ _____
Education	$ _____
Dues	$ _____
Gifts and donations	$ _____
Travel	$ _____
Subscriptions	$ _____
Automobile maintenance and gas	$ _____
Spending money and entertainment	$ _____

Food Expenses

Food—at home	$ _____
Food—away from home	$ _____

Taxes

Federal and state income tax	$ _____
Property	$ _____
Other taxes	$ _____

Other

Other	$ _____

TOTAL MONTHLY PAYMENTS $ _____

SAMPLE RECOMMENDED BUDGET EXPENDITURES

Shelter (rent or mortgage)	20%
Food	25%
Clothing	12%
Transportation	12%
Medical and dental	6%
Dues and charities	9%
Education and entertainment	10%
Savings	6%*

---

* Financial advisers recommend that savings should cover expenses for at least 3 months.

Figure 10-3

Chapter **10** **Basic Accounting and Finance**

1. Is having a budget useful? Why or why not?

_____

_____

_____

_____

_____

2. Do you consider savings an expense or income? Why?

_____

_____

_____

_____

_____

_____

3. List three expenses that are discretionary but necessary.

_____

_____

4. Explain why it is more (or less) expensive to eat in a restaurant than at home.

_____

_____

_____

5. What are two ways in which you could reduce your personal expenses without giving up discretionary expenditures that are important to you?

_____

_____

_____

_____

Capital Expenditures vs Operational, or Fixed, Expenditures

Capital expenditures are typically large, one-time expenses. Operational, or fixed, expenditures are routine expenses associated with everyday life.

1. What are some capital expenditures you have made? Large expenses are relative; you determine what constitutes a capital expenditure for yourself.

_____

_____

2. What are some operational, or fixed, expenditures in your life?

_____

_____

Payroll Projections

The healthcare organization plans yearly performance reviews and salary increases in September of each year. As the supervisor of the outpatient coding department, you are free to award raises as you see fit, but human resources has instructed department managers to limit the average of all raises in the department to 4%. The performance review ratings scale is as follows:

5 – Outstanding
4 – Exceeds Expectations
3 – Meets Expectations

2 – Needs Improvement

1 – Unacceptable

Your performance reviews have yielded the following scores for the department's employees:

Dot – 1.1

Pete – 2.9

Beth – 2.8

Roberta – 5.0

Using this information, how will you distribute raises? Assign each of your team members an increase in wages as your see fit based on the employee's performance, keeping in mind the 4% guidance from the organization. Note that it is possible to recommend that an employee's performance does not warrant a wage increase. Calculate the new salaries and complete the missing information in the table below.

Employee	Starting Annual Salary	August Monthly Pay	% Increase	Annual Salary Increase	New Annual Salary	September Monthly Pay
Dot	$35,000					
Pete	$36,000					
Beth	$30,000					
Roberta	$41,000					
Total	$142,000		Average increase must be ≤ 4%			

CRITICAL THINKING

Nonprofit Healthcare Providers

Many communities have free or reduced-cost healthcare services available through nonprofit organizations. Although the name would suggest otherwise, nonprofits actually do need to make money. The nonprofit designation means that an organization does not pay taxes; instead, it operates for the public good. Income above expense (net income) is reinvested in the organization.

1. Why do nonprofits need to make money?

2. If nonprofit healthcare services are provided at a lower cost, what are some strategies an organization might use to increase income and lower expenses in order to maintain a healthy balance sheet?

Payment Apps

A number of payment apps have become popular recently. Venmo, Zelle, PayPal and Cash App have changed the way people handle interpersonal transfers of money. Do you think these apps will eventually replace traditional banking? Why or why not?

_____

_____

_____

_____

_____

_____

_____

_____

11 Wellness, Growth, and Development

KNOWLEDGE CHECK

Multiple Choice

1. What is the optimal range of essential body fat for a female?
   a. 2–5%
   b. 10–13%
   c. 35–40%
   d. 55–59%

2. Which is **not** a measure of evaluating physical fitness?
   a. Balance
   b. Lung capacity
   c. Body fat percentage
   d. MRI or CT scan

3. Which method of *preventative health* involves managing a disease after the diagnosis has been made?
   a. Primary prevention
   b. Specified prevention
   c. Secondary prevention
   d. Tertiary prevention

4. Which level of *preventative health* may also be called a "screening"?
   a. Tertiary prevention
   b. Secondary prevention
   c. Primary prevention
   d. Specified prevention

5. Immunizations are included in which level of health prevention?
   a. Primary
   b. Secondary
   c. Tertiary
   d. Triage

6. Which is **not** a micronutrient?
   a. Vitamin B
   b. Calcium
   c. Protein
   d. Iron

7. What is the term for the amount of energy needed to raise 1 g of water by 1°C?
   a. Unit
   b. Catalyst
   c. Calorie
   d. Carbohydrate

8. The USDA introduced the food pyramid decades ago as a nutritional guide, and replaced it in 2011 with the
   a. MyKitchen model.
   b. MyFoods model.
   c. MyBody model.
   d. MyPlate model.

9. Water contains _____, a type of essential mineral.
   a. oxygen
   b. carbon
   c. lead
   d. electrolytes

10. The broad term for the many chemical reactions that occur in the body is
    a. nutrition.
    b. metabolism.
    c. defense mechanism.
    d. wellness.

11. Which nutrient aids in the manufacture of hormones?
    a. Protein
    b. Fat
    c. Carbohydrates
    d. Water

12. For a balanced diet, _____ of your daily calories should be from fats.
    a. 15%
    b. 55%
    c. 30%
    d. less than 10%

13. In the term *chronic stress*, the word chronic indicates an affliction that persists for
    a. 3 months or more.
    b. 1 month or more.
    c. 2 weeks or more.
    d. 6 months or more.

14. Endorphins are released by the brain during physical activity. What type of substances are endorphins?
    a. Vitamins
    b. Hormones
    c. Minerals
    d. Immune cells

15. In order to achieve cardiac benefits, experts say to raise the heart rate, or pulse, to about _____ of the maximum heart rate for 30 minutes, at least three times per week.
    a. 10%
    b. 25%
    c. 70%
    d. 100%

16. What is the meaning of the term *neonate*?
    a. Growth hormone contained in plasma
    b. The process of bone growth
    c. A baby from birth to 4 weeks old
    d. A mutation that stunts growth

17. Which age range makes up the young adult category?
    a. 8–13 years old
    b. 14–26 years old
    c. 30–39 years old
    d. 19–45 years old

18. According to psychiatrist Dr Elisabeth Kübler-Ross, during which of the five stages of grief might a person blame others for a loss?
    a. Acceptance
    b. Anger
    c. Denial
    d. Depression

19. Sanja, a health professional, is completing continuing education on the study of death, known as
    a. thanatology.
    b. expiration theory.
    c. sympathology.
    d. casualty studies.

20. A disease from which the patient is not expected to recover is called a(n)
    a. autonomous illness.
    b. palliative illness.
    c. terminal illness.
    d. acute illness.

Physical Well-Being

The textbook states that optimal wellness reflects a balanced relationship among a person's physical, mental, and social health.

1. Do you think your physical, mental, and social health are in a balanced relationship with each other? Why or why not?

_____

_____

_____

_____

_____

_____

2. Which area of your health would you like to strengthen: physical, mental, or social?

_____

_____

_____

_____

_____

_____

3. What is one thing you can do to strengthen that area?

_____

_____

_____

_____

_____

_____

Prevention

Provide three specific examples of each type of prevention: primary, secondary, and tertiary.

Type of Prevention	Examples (Three Each)
Primary	
Secondary	
Tertiary	

Nutrition

The USDA provides a tool, MyPlate, to help Americans learn more about healthful eating. Visit www.MyPlate.gov and take the quiz on the landing page. Then use one of the free resources and tools that follow completion of the quiz (MyPlate App, MyPlate Plan, or MyPlate Kitchen Recipes) to create a food plan and/or some food! If you choose to make one of the recipes, take a picture of the prepared dish to show your instructor.

Stress

Match the stress-related illness or disorder with the affected body system/body process.

_____ 1. Decreased attention	A. Muscular
_____ 2. Stomach ulcer	B. Skeletal
_____ 3. Arthritis	C. Cardiovascular
_____ 4. Increased infections	D. Digestive
_____ 5. Asthma	E. Psychosocial
_____ 6. Irritability	F. Endocrine
_____ 7. Backache	G. Respiratory
_____ 8. Angina	H. Immune
_____ 9. Diabetes	I. Nervous

Stress Management

Everyone experiences stress, and not all stress is bad. However, learning to manage stress will enables you to feel more in control of your emotions and decision-making abilities. Study Box 11-3, Stress Management Techniques, in the textbook. Choose one or two techniques to practice over the course of a week. Record your experiences in the table below.

Technique(s) Chosen:

1. _____

2. _____

Day	How I Used the Technique(s) Today
Monday	
Tuesday	
Wednesday	
Thursday	
Friday	
Saturday	
Sunday	

Exercise and Physical Activity

Physical activity benefits us on a number of levels. It can help reduce some factors that contribute to disease. And it is a mood booster. Without some level of activity, our muscles begin to atrophy (or muscle wasting) and our internal organs may not function properly.

1. Calculate your maximum heart rate (see Box 11-4 in the textbook). _____

2. Do you participate in physical activity that raises your heart rate to its maximum capacity (as calculated above) three times a week or more? _____

3. What are three benefits of physical activity that are meaningful to you?

    a. _____

    _____

    b. _____

    _____

    c. _____

    _____

4. If you are not currently exercising three times a week, what are the obstacles that prevent you from doing so?

    _____

    _____

    _____

    _____

5. Is there any exercise that you'd like to try if these obstacles could be overcome?

    _____

    _____

    _____

GROWTH AND DEVELOPMENT

Developmental Steps through the Life Span

For each developmental change write the stage of life in which it is first expected to occur.

Life Stages: Infant, Toddler, Preschooler, School-Age Child, Adolescent, Young Adult, Middle-age Adult, Older Adult

1. Establishes independence from family:_____

2. Earns most of the money and makes most of the decisions for society: _____

3. Peers become more important: _____

4. Needs constant care: _____

5. Accidents and respiratory illnesses are main threats to life: _____

6. Peers may assume primary importance: _____

7. Exhibits slower neurologic responses leading to slower sensory input interpretation:_____

8. Metabolic rate decreases: _____

9. Needs clear-cut rules: _____

10. Learns to speak: _____

11. Has uncontrolled motor responses: _____

Death and Dying

The textbook states that attitudes about death often change with circumstances and increased age, and that personal experience, religion, culture, and the ability to reason also determine a person's attitude about death. For this exercise, you will need to identify two people of widely different age, religion, culture, or personal experience to talk with. With consideration of the fact that death is a sensitive subject for many people, conduct a brief interview with each person. Possible questions are provided here, but you are free to ask your own. Write down your questions ahead of time, and make note of the answers you get. You may want to record the conversations (obtain permission first).

Potential Questions

1. Do you remember the first time you understood that someone or something died and would not return? How did you react?
2. What is more important to you, quality of life or length of life? Why?
3. What is your biggest fear about dying? How do you deal with that fear?
4. What are some of your religion's or culture's attitudes and beliefs about death? Do you agree with them?
5. Would you rather know you were going to die and therefore be able to plan and say your farewells, or would you rather die in your sleep or instantly in some other way?
6. What do you think happens to people after they die?
7. Have your attitudes about death changed over time?

After you have interviewed your subjects, answer these questions.

1. Why did you choose these two people?

_____

_____

_____

_____

2. What made them widely different from each other?

_____

_____

_____

_____

_____

3. Were their responses very different from each other's? If yes, how so?

_____

_____

_____

_____

4. What response surprised you most? Why?

_____

_____

_____

5. How did you feel asking questions about death?

_____

_____

_____

_____

6. Consider the questions you asked your subjects. What are your personal responses to those questions?

_____

_____

_____

_____

_____

_____

_____

_____

_____

_____

_____

_____

_____

_____

_____

_____

CRITICAL THINKING

Making the Decision to Die

In 1993, Michigan passed a law making assisted suicide a felony. This law resulted from the more than 17 assisted suicides involving Dr Jack Kevorkian. Groups that opposed Dr Kevorkian's actions questioned whether all of the suicides were actually voluntary.

When the Oregon Death with Dignity Act was passed in 1994, Oregon became the first state to legalize assisted suicide. However, the law was immediately challenged in the courts. This legislation allowed physicians to assist suicide in cases of terminal illness in which the life expectancy is 6 months or less. To obtain lethal medication under the law, the person must be diagnosed as terminally ill by at least two physicians. Groups that oppose the measure were concerned that people who are ill will choose to commit suicide to prevent expensive medical bills or to spare their loved ones from providing care for them.

87

In 1994, Benito Agrelo, a 15-year-old Florida boy, fought in court for the right to refuse a third transplant and medication. Benny had been born with a malfunctioning liver and had previously undergone two liver transplants. The drugs used to keep Benny's body from rejecting the liver caused migraine headaches and severe leg and back pain. Benny could not read or walk. Benny's physicians felt that he could be helped by a third transplant and a change in the dosage of the immunosuppressive medication. Using the child abuse agencies and laws, the physicians forced Benny to return to the hospital. After hearings with a judge, Benny was allowed to return home and refuse treatment. Benny stopped taking the medication and died in August 1994. Before he died, he reported that those last months were the best months of his life.

In 2006, 16-year-old Abraham Cherrix went to court in Virginia to win the right to refuse chemotherapy for treatment of Hodgkin disease, a type of blood cancer. Abraham had been previously treated with chemotherapy but chose to follow an alternative treatment when the disease recurred. His parents were charged with medical negligence. In August 2006, charges against his parents were dropped when Abraham agreed to treatment by an oncologist who is supportive of the alternative medicine approach.

In 2021, eight states have enacted *physician-assisted dying* or *aid-in-dying* laws. In these states, mentally competent adults with 6 or fewer months to live may obtain a prescription from a physician that will end their lives when administered.

1. In your opinion, is it suicide for a person to refuse treatment, as Abraham did, or medication, as in the case of Benny? Why or why not?

2. In your opinion, should someone who is terminally ill be allowed to end his or her life? Why or why not?

3. If you gave a positive response to Question 2, who do you think should be involved in a decision to end someone's life?

4. In your opinion, what gives a person's life value?

_____

_____

_____

_____

_____

_____

_____

_____

12 Safety and Health Practices

KNOWLEDGE CHECK

Multiple Choice

Circle the one correct answer to each of the following questions.

1. What is the name for the series of events that leads to a microbe to cause an infection?
   a. Consequence of infection
   b. Chain of infection
   c. Chain of causation
   d. Infection causation

2. An infection requires a _____ in which the microorganisms will grow and reproduce.
   a. portal
   b. reservoir
   c. host
   d. fomite

3. What is the correct medical term for a contagious disease?
   a. Transferrable disease
   b. Passing disease
   c. Moveable disease
   d. Communicable disease

4. Which of these is a type of infectious microbe?
   a. Fungi
   b. Protein
   c. Cholesterol
   d. Lead

5. What is the term for the habitat where the infectious organism usually lives, grows, and multiplies?
   a. Carrier
   b. Portal
   c. Microbiome
   d. Reservoir

6. A person with an infection that is otherwise healthy and has shown no signs of the infection is called a
   a. convalescent carrier.
   b. chronic carrier.
   c. passive carrier.
   d. incubatory carrier.

7. What is the term for the type of carrier who can infect another person after they have recovered from the illness themselves?
   a. Convalescent carrier
   b. Chronic carrier
   c. Passive carrier
   d. Incubatory carrier

8. Which is a direct contact mode of transmission for infections?
   a. Aerosol
   b. Oral
   c. Vehicle
   d. Vector

9. Living intermediaries, such as other humans, are called
   a. vectors.
   b. vehicles.
   c. microbes.
   d. aerosols.

10. Edith went to the ER with chills, pain, and all over discomfort accompanied by a fever. She was told she has an infection. Which type of infection does Edith likely have?
    a. A local infection
    b. A universal infection
    c. A systemic infection
    d. A minor infection

11. What is the acronym for the common hospital infection that is often referred to as a "superbug" due to its resistance to antibiotics?
    a. SARS
    b. SMAR
    c. MARS
    d. MRSA

12. Standard Precautions are infection prevention techniques that are applied to
    a. a random sample of patients.
    b. infected patients.
    c. patients suspected of infection disease (but not confirmed).
    d. all patients regardless of diagnosis.

13. Which precautions are applied to patients who are suspected of having an infection?
    a. Transmission-Based
    b. Universal
    c. Standard
    d. Special

14. The term for the absence of any disease-causing microbes is known as
    a. sanitized.
    b. decontaminated.
    c. clean.
    d. aseptic.

15. What is the name of the equipment that uses pressurized steam to sterilize materials?
    a. Ethylene oxide unit
    b. Reservoir
    c. Vector
    d. Autoclave

16. After applying soap, what is the minimum amount of time the health care professional should rub the hands while performing handwashing?
    a. 20 seconds
    b. 1 minute
    c. 10 seconds
    d. 3 seconds

17. What is the meaning of the medical term *zoonosis*?
    a. The testing of treatments on animals, prior to testing on humans
    b. The studying of animals
    c. An infectious disease transmissible from animals to humans, under normal conditions
    d. A grouping technique for studying viruses

18. The agency within the Department of Labor that establishes and enforces workplace safety standards is the
    a. Workplace Health and Safety Commission.
    b. Occupational Safety and Health Administration.
    c. American Human Resources Administration.
    d. Occupational Workplace Safety Commission.

19. What is the meaning of the term ergonomics?
    a. Financial calculations to find out the cost to train employees about safety
    b. The practice of keeping an organized workspace
    c. The design of the workplace to maximize comfort and productivity
    d. The fiscal cost of creating a safe work environment
20. Female nurses are about twice as likely to experience back problems as females in other professions. A device that provides _____ can help, specifically in preventing back injuries.
    a. warmth, such as warmer clothes
    b. postural support, such as a brace
    c. balance, such as quality footwear
    d. compression, such as joint braces
21. According to the fire plan acronym RACE, what does the "E" stand for?
    a. Enter
    b. Extradite
    c. Extinguish
    d. Everyone
22. The third step in the RACE fire emergency protocol, after *alarm*, is
    a. Confine or contain
    b. Coworkers or co-inhabitants
    c. Correct or corrective
    d. Counter or counteract
23. When discharging a fire extinguisher, the P.A.S.S. technique should be used. What does this acronym stand for?
    a. Press, air, squeeze, separate
    b. Pause, aim, swarm, sweep
    c. Pull, aim, squeeze, sweep
    d. Press, air, squeeze, surround
24. Medical waste is either general medical waste or biohazardous waste. Which of these is **not** considered biohazardous waste?
    a. Sharps
    b. Human tissue
    c. Debris swept up from patient's room floor
    d. Supplies that may be contaminated

DISEASE TRANSMISSION

Pathogenic or Infectious Agents
Match the type of microorganism with the disease it causes. Use (V) Virus, (B) Bacteria, (F) Fungus, (P) Protozoa, and (W) Worms.

_____ 1. Influenza

_____ 2. Tetanus

_____ 3. Gonorrhea

_____ 4. Hepatitis B

_____ 5. Elephantiasis

_____ 6. Malaria

_____ 7. Vaginal yeast infection

_____ 8. Mumps

_____ 9. Rabies

Chain of Infection

In order for infection to occur, a specific set of elements must interact in a specific sequence. This interaction is called the chain of infection. Choose a pathogen to move through the chain of infection. Use your creativity to illustrate the journey of this pathogen. You can draw, use images from print or online media, or even write a short story describing the pathogen's movement along the chain of infection.

Zoonosis

Non-human animals are able to transmit some diseases, or zoonoses, to humans, and vice versa. Choose a zoonotic disease to research (the CDC website is a good resource for this). Share your findings by answering these questions.

1. What disease did you research?

_____

2. Which animal(s) most commonly transmit it?

_____

3. Where in the world is the disease most prevalent?

_____

4. What is the prevalence rate in the United States?

_____

5. What are some precautions to take to avoid infection with the pathogen?

_____

_____

6. What is the treatment for this disease?

_____

_____

Mode of Transmission

Modes of disease transmission are classified as direct or indirect contact transmission. For each mode of transmission, list an example of a pathogen (not already found in Chapter 12) and give an example of how it is transmitted by that mode.

Mode of Transmission	Pathogen	Example
Direct contact		
Oral (direct contact)		
Aerosol (indirect contact)		
Vehicle (indirect contact)		
Vector (indirect contact)		

Local vs Systemic vs Asymptomatic Infection

Infection may involve many signs and symptoms, or none, and may occur in a small, localized area, or spread throughout the body. For each scenario described, what is the most likely type of infection: local, systemic, or asymptomatic?

Scenario	Probable Type of Infection (Local, Systemic, Asymptomatic)
Yesterday, Tina stepped on a new thumb tack that had fallen out of the family calendar in the kitchen. The tiny puncture mark in her heel is sore and a little bit red.	
Silas's teammate tested positive for COVID-19, so the whole team had to get tested. To Silas's surprise, his test came back positive, even though he has felt fine and hadn't missed a practice all season.	
Cena is really regretting her decision to eat the leftover shrimp scampi she found in the fridge. She *thought* it was her husband's from his meal out last night, but now she's guessing it was actually her daughter's from the previous weekend. Cena has been vomiting all day, and has a fever, aches, and chills.	
Jim has the flu; the doctor confirmed it. He can't even lie on the couch to watch TV. He just has to go to bed with the lights out. He's sweating so much he knows he'll have to change the sheets before morning.	
Sophie has felt this sensation before: she has to urinate frequently, and when she does, it really stings! She calls her nurse practitioner and asks for antibiotics. "It's a UTI, I'm sure of it," Sophie tells the nurse.	

Precautions

Read the following statements and write "T" for true or "F" for false in the blanks provided. If a statement is false, correct the statement to make it true.

1. The primary method of infection prevention is PPE.
2. Universal precautions are broader than Standard Precautions.
3. Feces, nasal secretions, sputum, tears, urine, and vomitus are not considered reason to use Universal Precautions, unless those substances also contain visible blood.
4. The three categories of Transmission-Based Precautions guidelines are airborne, indirect, and contact precautions.
5. Hands that have been protected by sterile gloves do not require washing after removal of the gloves.
6. PPE stands for personal protective equipment, such as gloves and masks.
7. Prevention of injury from needles, scalpels, and other sharps is the major purpose of Transmission-Based Precautions.
8. Contact precautions are used for infections spread through the air, such as chickenpox.

Principles of Asepsis

Match each characteristic with the level of medical asepsis with which it is associated: antiseptic, disinfectant, or sterile.

Characteristic	Level of Asepsis (Antiseptic, Disinfectant, or Sterile)
Can be used on the skin	
Is often accomplished by autoclave	
The removal of all microorganisms	
Can be accomplished by boiling	
Inhibits the growth of bacteria, but does not necessarily kill it	

Osha

Review Box 12-2, Common Workplace Hazards. For each type of hazard listed, choose one and indicate a situation in which a healthcare professional might encounter it. Please choose a different type of healthcare professional for each example. An example has been provided.

Type of Hazard (choose one from each type)	Career Impacted	Example
Mechanical: Impact	Nurse	A nurse slips on a recently washed floor in the hospital hallway
Mechanical:		
Physical:		
Biological:		
Chemical:		
Psychosocial:		

Safety Data Sheets

Review Box 12-3, Safety Data Sheet (SDS). Prepare a list of the SDS requirements for a common household item on a note card, excluding the name of the product. Compare and trade cards with classmates. Use the information to identify as many of the products as possible.

1. Which household items were you able to identify using the SDS information?

_____

_____

_____

2. Were any of the household items more or less dangerous than you expected?

_____

_____

3. Based on the information in the SDS cards, will you use any of the products differently?

_____

_____

_____

Body Mechanics and Ergonomics

Research correct body mechanics and ergonomics for two activities you probably spend a lot of time doing as a student: sitting at a desk and using a smart phone.

Correct body mechanics for sitting at a desk:

_____

_____

_____

_____

_____

Correct body mechanics for using a smart phone:

_____

_____

_____

_____

_____

Fire and Electrical Hazards

Create a pamphlet or PowerPoint presentation that illustrates the concepts of "RACE" and "PASS" in the school or health care facility setting. The pamphlet should be designed to educate the reader about these concepts. It should include emergency exits, equipment, and phone numbers that are appropriate to the facility chosen.

EMERGENCY PREPAREDNESS

Three Days

Box 12-5 lists items to include in an emergency kit for 3 days. Discuss the list with the people with whom you live, and collect the items if possible to have on hand. This exercise is simply for your benefit.

CRITICAL THINKING

Case Studies

For each scenario, describe an appropriate response.

1. While providing care for a patient, you find that someone has left an uncapped needle on the bedside tray. What should you do?

_____

_____

_____

_____

2. You are using Transmission-Based Precautions to care for a patient. When it is completed, you notice that one of your gloves has ripped sometime during the care. What should you do?

_____

_____

_____

_____

3. As part of his daily care, you need to help an obese patient move from the bed to a chair. You ask one of your co-workers to help you. She responds that she moves that man by herself every day. What should you do?

_____

_____

_____

_____

4. You are providing daily care for a patient and find a lighter and cigarettes in the bedside drawer. What should you do?

_____

_____

_____

_____

13 Professionalism and Effective Communication

KNOWLEDGE CHECK

Multiple Choice

Circle the one correct answer to each of the following questions.

1. Employers like applicants with both hard skills and soft skills. What is an example of a soft skill?
   a. Medical coding
   b. Keyboarding/typing
   c. Being responsible
   d. CPR certification

2. Healthcare professionals with higher emotional intelligence (EI) will have a better understanding of
   a. the rules.
   b. their position.
   c. their feelings.
   d. their employer's business model.

3. What is the name for a measure of emotional intelligence?
   a. Emotional formula
   b. Emotional quotient
   c. Emotion map
   d. Emotion bar

4. Which term means the quality of being honest and having strong principles?
   a. Dependable
   b. Integrity
   c. Responsibility
   d. Reciprocity

5. Someone is described as dependable when they show _____ behavior.
   a. consistent
   b. unusual
   c. polite
   d. positive

6. Research has shown that _____ makes up 70–80% of communication.
   a. verbal communication
   b. gossip
   c. vocabulary
   d. nonverbal communication

7. Which skill involves giving full attention to the speaker, including body language?
   a. Nonverbal communication
   b. Active listening
   c. Brainstorming
   d. Organization

8. Which statement about professional writing is correct?
   a. The more words, the better.
   b. Professionals use the longest words they can.
   c. It is important to consider the reader.
   d. The most essential information should go in the last sentence.

9. Which communication tool involves using encouraging words with nonverbal cues?
   a. Reflecting
   b. Questioning
   c. Reinforcement
   d. Active listening

10. Which communication tool is a good technique to draw someone into a conversation?
   a. Reflecting
   b. Questioning
   c. Reinforcement
   d. Active listening

11. A(n) _____ position is usually the first one a person obtains after completing his or her training.
   a. supervisory
   b. clinical
   c. internship
   d. entry-level

12. In healthcare, you will interact with many people, most importantly
   a. coworkers.
   b. friends.
   c. supervisors.
   d. patients.

13. Which method is effective for increasing your vocabulary?
   a. Reading material you are already familiar with
   b. Limiting sleep
   c. Using a "Word of the Day" app
   d. Watching cartoons

14. Research shows that reading as little as _____ will help grow your vocabulary.
   a. 5 hours a day
   b. 1 minute a day
   c. 1 hour a week
   d. 20 minutes a day

15. The _____ of your voice includes both speed and volume.
   a. tone
   b. pitch
   c. sound
   d. rhythm

PROFESSIONALISM

Identifying Professional Behaviors

1. Jennifer Lynelle is a registered nurse who works in the ICU of a mid-sized hospital in Denver. Although Denver is infamous for its snowfall and unpredictable weather, Jennifer has never been late to work! She knows that she has to plan ahead by keeping her car in good condition for winter driving, and allowing extra time for travel on days when the weather will be bad.
   What aspect(s) of professionalism is Jennifer practicing?

2. Ramesh Puri is a phlebotomy technician in a diagnostics laboratory outside of Philadelphia. He spends most of his time at work drawing blood samples from patients who bring in orders from their physicians. Some days are incredibly busy, with scheduled and walk-in patients packing the waiting and exam rooms. On a particularly harried day, Ramesh realizes he has forgotten to label one of the tubes he used for a draw. He is almost positive the sample belongs to Mr Shaw, the patient he saw right before Ms Jimenez. But he cannot be 100% sure because he had not affixed the label at the time of the draw. Ramesh immediately tells his supervisor what he has done.
   What aspect(s) of professionalism is Ramesh displaying?

3. Susanne Brown is a social worker at a clinic for migrant farmworkers in rural Georgia. Most of the clients she sees are from Central and South America. Susanne is fluent in Spanish, and she enjoys being able to communicate with this population. She loves to see the relief so many of her clients feel when they realize they are understood. Recently, however, a significant number of new clients have come to the clinic from Belle Glade, FL. They are originally from

Haiti, and they speak Creole. Susanne recognizes that she needs to use the services of Tamara Jean-Louis, the clinic's newly hired Creole interpreter.

What aspect(s) of professionalism is Susanne exhibiting?

_____

EMOTIONAL INTELLIGENCE

Ideally, all healthcare professionals would possess a high level of professionalism and emotional intelligence. Healthcare professionals with higher emotional intelligence have a better understanding of their emotions and how to manage them in themselves and in others, which is an essential skill when interacting with patients.

Many resources are available to help you better understand emotional intelligence and improve your own emotional quotient (EQ). One source is https://www.helpguide.org/articles/mental-health/emotional-intelligence-eq.htm, which describes the components of emotional intelligence (EI) and how to improve key skills. By researching EI on that website or another source, identify a component of EI that you would like to increase in yourself. Describe the aspect of EI that you would benefit from working on, and list three ways to improve it.

Measure of EI to improve:

_____

Ways to improve:

_____
_____
_____
_____
_____
_____
_____
_____
_____

EMPLOYER EXPECTATIONS

Box 13-1 in the textbook lists common expectations of employers for employees. It is not an all-inclusive list. Think of at least two other reasonable expectations that an employer would have of an employee.

_____
_____
_____
_____
_____

JOB READINESS

Job Readiness Skills Self-Assessment

Box 13-4 in the textbook delineates job readiness skills and attributes. Think about your own potential readiness for a job. You may already have a job, you may be seeking one, or you may be thinking in terms of the period after graduation from your last year of formal education. Give an example from your life when you have demonstrated each skill. If you do not have any evidence of possessing that skill, think of a way you might develop it.

Skill	Current Example	Potential Development
Having integrity, honesty, loyalty		
Good communication skills		
Time management		
Teamwork and collaboration skills		
Ability to do presentations		
Confidence		
Having a strong work ethic		
Flexibility and adaptability		
Leadership and ability to take initiative		
Ability to manage stress		
Patience and empathy for others		

EFFECTIVE COMMUNICATION

Nonverbal Communication

Nonverbal communication is a form communication where we send and receive messages without using our verbal communication skills. Nonverbal communication includes facial expressions, the tone of voice, eye contact, and body language gestures. Research has shown that nonverbal communication makes up 70–80% of communication. Understanding nonverbal communication is an important component of both expression and reception of messages.

Think about your own experiences with nonverbal communication. List three nonverbal behaviors that suggest a listener is paying attention, and three that suggest inattention or distraction.

Attention	Inattention

The Right Word

It is important to use correct grammar, spelling, and word choice when writing or speaking professionally. Circle the sentence in each pair that has correct grammar, spelling, and word choice.

1. Dr Miller has saw 32 patients in the emergency room tonight.
2. Dr Miller has seen 32 patients in the emergency room tonight.
1. Affective communication is critical to success in the workplace.
2. Effective communication is critical to success in the workplace.
1. Melinda is experienced at inserting intravenous catheters.
2. Melinda is experienced at inserting intraveinous catheters.
1. Massage therapy is a growing occupation.
2. Massage therapy is a growing occupation.
1. The human resources representative selected the continuing education courses for Tina and me.
2. The human resources representative selected the continuing education courses for Tina and I.

Building Vocabulary

A simple practice to increase vocabulary is to use a "word-a-day" application. If you have a smart phone, download such an app (there are multiple free versions). Practice using the new words each day.

CRITICAL THINKING

Integrity

"Integrity is a keystone of personal and professional success."
Do you agree with this assertion? Why or why not?

_____

_____

_____

_____

_____

_____

Do you think integrity is more important for healthcare professionals than for people in other professions? Why or why not?

_____

_____

_____

_____

_____

_____

_____

Chapter **13** **Professionalism and Effective Communication**

Who in your life demonstrates a high level of integrity? What behaviors indicate their integrity?

_____

_____

_____

_____

_____

_____

_____

_____

_____

_____

_____

_____

_____

_____

_____

Multiple Choice

Circle the one correct answer to each of the following questions.

1. What is the term for a preconceived notion or generalized opinion about a group or situation that often serves as a mental shortcut to classify others?
   a. Conscious bias
   b. Prejudice
   c. Unconscious bias
   d. Stereotype

2. Prejudices are feelings, opinions, or ideas based on
   a. reasoning.
   b. facts.
   c. personal perception.
   d. cultural competency.

3. Which kind of bias exists when a person's attitudes and related behaviors are clear and whose biased actions are conducted intentionally?
   a. Conscious bias
   b. Direct bias
   c. Abnormal bias
   d. Unconscious bias

4. The differences among people on the job is referred to as
   a. discrimination.
   b. workplace diversity.
   c. occupational bias.
   d. cultural competence.

5. A hiring manager offers a Hispanic applicant work in the hospital's environmental services instead of the pharmacy because most of the employees in environmental services are Hispanic. This is an example of
   a. cultural competence.
   b. bias.
   c. stereotyping.
   d. discrimination.

6. In what year did the U.S. Supreme Court determine it was illegal to fire an employee for being gay or transgender?
   a. 1990
   b. 1965
   c. 2020
   d. 1975

7. Which government agency enforces anti-discrimination laws?
   a. The U.S. Department of Commerce
   b. The U.S. Treasury Department
   c. The U.S. Equal Employment Opportunity Commission
   d. The Federal Trade Commission

8. Members of some cultures will not take cough syrup because it contains which substance?
   a. Alcohol
   b. Olive oil
   c. Caffeine
   d. Ginger

9. Part of Title VI of the Civil Rights Act requires healthcare facilities to provide a(n) _____ to patients who speak limited or no English.
    a. rebate
    b. discount
    c. translator
    d. bilingual physician

10. A pregnant patient explains to her OB/GYN that her grandmother believes she should not go out at night because the baby could be harmed if a pregnant woman is exposed to moonlight. However, the patient says she does not hold this belief and will continue to work the night shift. What is the term for the patient's embrace of the dominant culture?
    a. Prejudice
    b. Bias
    c. Acculturation
    d. Cultural competency

11. In 1967, the Age Discrimination in Employment Act (ADEA) was passed protecting employees over which age from discrimination in the workplace?
    a. 50
    b. 40
    c. 65
    d. 55

12. What is the term for a practice that a culture forbids, believing it will bring on a negative consequence?
    a. Taboo
    b. Jargon
    c. Rite
    d. Ritual

13. Prior to _____, making public places accessible to people with disabilities was not mandated by law.
    a. 1945
    b. 2015
    c. 1885
    d. 1990

14. What is the term for the skills required to ensure quality of patient care and equality in healthcare?
    a. Unconscious bias
    b. Cultural competence
    c. Workplace diversity
    d. Discrimination avoidance

15. Which of these cultural groups forbids the mixing of meat and dairy?
    a. Asian
    b. Native American
    c. Jewish
    d. Hispanic

16. In which of these cultures is alcohol forbidden?
    a. Muslim
    b. Asian
    c. Jewish
    d. Native American

True/False

Read the following statements and write "T" for true or "F" for false in the blanks provided. If a statement is false, correct the statement to make it true.

_____ 1. Many cultures have preferences about foods.

_____ 2. Another term for conscious bias is implicit bias.

_____ 3. Tamir is a nurse who is communicating with a patient who does not speak English. He is correct in making sure to speak to the interpreter directly, not the patient.

_____ 4. Some stereotypes, such as that Asians are good at math, are positive and therefore are helpful.

_____ 5. Race, gender, sexual orientation, even a person's weight are all characteristics subject to bias.

_____ 6. Employers that do not recruit from diverse talent pools will see a decrease in hiring costs.

_____ 7. It is legal for a potential employer to ask job candidates if they have children, but not whether they have childcare available.

_____ 8. Individualism and autonomy are generally values of western healthcare culture.
_____ 9. Culture influences behaviors like eating habits, choice of clothing, and hobbies.
_____ 10. Both federal and state laws exist to protect workers from discrimination.

CULTURE

Cultural Influences in Our Lives

Write two brief paragraphs about how your own culture has influenced you in two of the areas mentioned in the textbook.

1. Area of cultural influence:_____
   Influence in my life:

_____

_____

_____

_____

_____

_____

2. Area of cultural influence:_____
   Influence in my life:

_____

_____

_____

_____

_____

_____

STEREOTYPES, PREJUDICES, AND BIASES

Examining Our Own Beliefs

Stereotypes, prejudices, and biases come from many sources, and all people have some. Consider some of your views that meet the definition of stereotypes, prejudices, and biases. Think about where they originated: family, friends, media, etc. What have you done or can you do to challenge them?

1. Stereotype, prejudice, or bias

_____

_____

_____

2. Where did this idea come from?

_____

_____

_____

_____

Chapter **14** **Cultural Competence and Workplace Diversity**

3. What have you done or could you do to challenge this view?

_____

_____

_____

_____

Personal Experience with Stereotypes, Prejudices, and Biases

As discussed, stereotyping, prejudice, and bias are universal experiences of human beings. It is likely that at some point, you have been the subject of someone else's stereotype, prejudice, or bias. Can you think of an instance when that happened? How did you feel? Were your internal and external reactions different? Write about your experience.

_____

_____

_____

_____

_____

_____

_____

_____

_____

_____

_____

_____

WORKPLACE DIVERSITY

Benefits of Workplace Diversity

Box 14-3 lists benefits of workplace diversity in your textbook. Provide an example of, or rationale for, each.

Benefit	Example or Rationale
Improves creativity	
Improves productivity and profits	
Improves employee engagement and employee retention	
Increases range of skills and knowledge	
Expands talent pool and attracts more candidates	

Employee Discrimination Laws

Employment laws have been enacted over the last several decades to ensure that applying for a job, hiring, maintaining a job, and managing employees are activities that take place without discrimination. Read the following synopses of employment discrimination laws. Then, indicate the name of the law, and the year it was passed.

Purpose	Name of Law	Year of Passage
Prohibits discrimination of the basis of pregnancy, childbirth, and/or a medical condition related to pregnancy or childbirth		
Requires that the individual receives "reasonable" accommodations, if necessary, and should not be discriminated against in the pursuit of employment, education, or access to public places because of disability		
Prohibits wage differentials based on sex		
Protects employees or future employees who are 40 or older from discrimination in the workplace		
Makes it illegal to discriminate against someone on the basis of race, color, religion, national origin or sex. This law also protects employees against retaliation for going forward with a claim regarding discrimination in the workplace		
Prohibited discrimination against a job applicant or an employee during a variety of work situations including hiring, firing, promotions, training, wages and benefits		

Employment Discrimination Law History

Research one of the laws discussed in Section 14.4.2. Find out when the legislation was initially introduced. Who supported it, and why? Who opposed it, and why?

Law: _____

Year legislation introduced: _____

Support: _____

_____

_____

_____

_____

_____

_____

Opposition: _____

_____

_____

_____

_____

_____

CULTURAL COMPETENCE IN HEALTHCARE

Cultural competence entails understanding, valuing, and taking into account the traditions, norms, and beliefs of other cultures when interacting with members of those cultures. It also means staying abreast of current information about differences in the actions and side effects of medications and treatments based on patient ethnicity. Using an interpreter so that communication is clear is also an integral part of cultural competence. It is not always easy to develop and use cultural competence as a healthcare provider, but it is critical to your patients. Cultural competence can have a significant impact on health outcomes. Box 14-7 in the textbook details some skills for building cultural competency.

109

When Epilepsy Goes By Another Name

The Spirit Catches You and You Fall Down is the story of a Hmong family's interaction with Western medicine in the care and treatment of a child with epilepsy. The author of the book, Anne Fadiman, describes the challenges for both the family and their doctors in attempting to care for and treat the child. Read an interview with the author on the Epilepsy Foundation website: https://www.epilepsy.com/article/2014/3/when-epilepsy-goes-another-name.

1. How does the author describe the view of epilepsy in the Hmong people?

_____

_____

_____

_____

_____

_____

2. What does the author think is the most important lesson for doctors to take away from this story?

_____

_____

_____

_____

_____

_____

Using an Interpreter

Culturally and linguistically appropriate services (CLAS) is a term that refers to the implementation and use of cultural competence in healthcare. Visit the U.S. Department of Health and Human Services Think Cultural Health website (https://thinkculturalhealth.hhs.gov/). Listen to the In Your Words video under Testimonials.

1. Imagine you are a direct provider of healthcare and you are working with someone whose language you do not speak or understand. After watching this video, explain the significance of using an interpreter rather than a family member to communicate with your patient.

_____

_____

_____

_____

_____

_____

_____

15 Employment and Career Development

KNOWLEDGE CHECK

Multiple Choice

Circle the one correct answer to each of the following questions.

1. What is the name for the standard group of healthcare skills, created by the National Consortium on Health Science and Technology?
   a. National Healthcare Techniques List
   b. Core and Cluster Skill Set
   c. National Nursing Skill Standards
   d. National Healthcare Skill Standards

2. Time management is an important healthcare job skill that involves the organization of a(n)
   a. portfolio.
   b. schedule.
   c. language.
   d. application.

3. Essential supporting skills such as communication, problem-solving, and accepting responsibility are considered
   a. soft skills.
   b. unconscious skills.
   c. implicit skills.
   d. hard skills.

4. What is the name for the specialized form of documenting notes on medical records?
   a. Prospecting
   b. Visualizing
   c. Charting
   d. Shorting

5. The type of résumé that emphasizes skills and traits pulled from work and personal experiences relating to a targeted job opening is called a _____ résumé.
   a. chronological
   b. functional
   c. combination
   d. traditional

6. A chronological résumé lists an applicant's prior jobs in what order?
   a. From highest paying to least paying
   b. From oldest to newest
   c. From most recent to oldest
   d. From most relevant to the job to least relevant.

7. What is the name for a business letter that describes how and why you are a good fit for a specific job?
   a. Portfolio
   b. Reference list
   c. Résumé
   d. Cover letter

8. "Designed," "generated," and "chosen" are all examples of
   a. descriptors.
   b. starters.
   c. power words.
   d. visualizing words.

9. A collection of your work samples and achievements to show a prospective employer is called a
   a. power folder.
   b. cover letter.
   c. functional résumé.
   d. portfolio.
10. Which of these is **not** a technique to answer behavioral interview questions?
    a. STAR
    b. PAR
    c. START
    d. SHARE
11. Ben has an interview tomorrow morning but does not know what to wear. He cannot reach the office to ask. What should Ben wear?
    a. Button-down shirt and jeans
    b. A two-piece suit
    c. A sweater, nice jeans, and dress shoes
    d. Jeans, a t-shirt, and tennis shoes
12. Jen is preparing for an interview using the videoconferencing app Zoom. What kind of interview is this?
    a. Multimedia
    b. Phone
    c. Traditional
    d. Virtual
13. Illegal interview questions such as those about an applicant's race, political affiliation, sexual orientation, or gender identity are forbidden based on the guidelines of
    a. the U.S. Department of Commerce (DOC).
    b. the employer's HR department.
    c. the U.S. Equal Employment Opportunity Commission (EEOC).
    d. the American Civil Liberties Union (ACLU).
14. A job offer should not be considered official unless it is presented
    a. in person.
    b. over the phone.
    c. through another employee.
    d. in writing.
15. What is the term for training and study that is completed after the worker begins to practice in the profession?
    a. Continuing education
    b. Extended studies
    c. Advanced education
    d. Work study
16. Which is a common form of retirement plan where taxes are deferred until age 59½?
    a. 401(k)
    b. 140(k)
    c. 410(k)
    d. 410(j)
17. It is not recommended to discuss salary until
    a. the second interview.
    b. a job offer is made to you.
    c. the end of your first day of work.
    d. you have accepted the position.

True/False

Read the following statements and write "T" for true or "F" for false in the blanks provided. If a statement is false, correct the statement to make it true.

_____1. Mary is into fashion and posts many photos on social media sites. Her parents think many of the photos are provocative. It is possible that an employer will see this content and be dissuaded from hiring her, as it does not demonstrate professionalism. Mary should consider removing photos or comments that do not portray a professional candidate.

_____2. Although time management and communication are important skills in the working world, test-taking and note-taking are no longer relevant once you have finished school.

_____3. Soft skills are important in sales and politics, but have little application in the provision of healthcare.

_____ 4. On average, approximately one-third of life is spent working.

_____ 5. Job search activities including preparing a skills inventory, writing a résumé, and putting together a support team.
_____ 6. You should avoid the use of personal pronouns such as I, me, or my when writing your résumé.
_____ 7. A combination résumé is usually the best option for a person just entering the job market.
_____ 8. It is important to keep an open mind and not research a potential employer prior to an interview.
_____ 9. Establishing expected compensation is a critical component of the initial interview.
_____ 10. Employee benefits can represent a significant portion of your compensation.

EMPLOYMENT

Standard Skills for Healthcare Professionals

Box 15-2 in the textbook lists a number of standard skills for healthcare professionals. Complete the table with explanations and/or examples of basic professional standards for each of the following factors.

Factor	Standard
Hygiene	
Clothing	
Language	
Confidentiality	
Behavior	

CAREER DEVELOPMENT

Examining Expectations

1. Each person seeks different things from a job. Consider what you would like to experience and gain from your employment. Write a paragraph about your expectations for the short- and long-term views of your career.
   a. Short-term expectations

   _____
   _____
   _____
   _____
   _____
   _____

   b. Long-term expectations

   _____
   _____
   _____
   _____
   _____
   _____
   _____
   _____

113

2. Ask a working person in your life about his or her expectations of work. The person does not have to be a healthcare professional, just someone with whom you feel comfortable discussing this.

a. What were the expectations for the job or career when he or she was just entering the workforce?

_____

_____

_____

_____

_____

_____

_____

b. Have those expectations been met? How or how not?

_____

_____

_____

_____

_____

_____

_____

c. What advice would this person offer you for starting your career?

_____

_____

_____

_____

_____

_____

Portfolio Preparation

Assemble a portfolio following link to the HOSA criteria:

http://www.hosa.org/sites/default/files/Health%20Science%20Portfolio.pdf

_____ Letter of introduction

_____ Résumé

_____ Project description

_____ Writing sample

_____ Work-based learning

_____ Oral presentation

_____ Service learning

_____ Credentials

_____ Technology

_____ Leadership experience

Mock Interview

Choose a partner with whom to practice an interview. Think about the employer and the position for which the interview is being held. For example, the employer might be the local pharmacy manager, and the position could be the pharmacy assistant (or technician). Or an orthopedic physicians' practice might be interviewing candidates for a physical therapist position. Be creative and specific. Use Box 15-2 in the textbook for suggestions for questions to include in the process. Then switch roles.

Thank You Note

After your mock interview, write a brief thank you note to the "interviewer," thanking him or her for the opportunity and summarizing your qualifications.

_____

_____

_____

_____

_____

_____

_____

_____

Behavioral Interview

Practice your own behavioral interview. Using Box 15-13 in the textbook, choose the SHARE, STAR, or PAR model. Think of a situation, problem, or task you have encountered, and use your chosen model to answer the questions associated with it. Construct answers that demonstrate your capabilities. Get bonus points for using "power" words! (See Table 15-2 in the textbook.)

S *or* **S** *or* **P**	
H *or* **T** *or* **A**	
A *or* **A** *or* **R**	
P *or* **R**	
E	

Evaluating the Job Offer

The candidate you interviewed for the job in Section 15.4.1, Mock Interview, is the best-qualified applicant! Acting as the employer, write a job offer for the candidate that includes the pertinent information as outlined in the textbook. Highlight or circle each of those pieces of information.

_____

_____

_____

_____

_____

_____

_____

_____

_____

_____

_____

_____

_____

_____

_____

_____

Employee Benefits

Using the Internet and/or other resources, research the range of costs for each of these potential employee benefits for the health career that interests you most.

Benefit	Cost Range
Individual health insurance	
Continuing education	
Uniforms (if applicable)	
Professional association dues	
Student loan repayment	

What Matters Most

People want different things from work: money, prestige, meaning, etc. What are the three most important things you would like to obtain from your job or career? Why?

_____

_____

_____

_____

_____

_____

_____

_____

Thinking Ahead

In Section 15.3.1, you wrote about your long-term expectations for your career. What are some steps you can take now that will help you meet those expectations? What are some actions you should avoid in order to have a better chance of meeting your career goals?

_____

_____

_____

_____

_____

_____

_____

_____

_____

16 Academic Foundation

Multiple Choice

1. Organization is directly related to
   a. personality.
   b. self-esteem.
   c. efficiency.
   d. mistakes.

2. When someone decides what is urgent versus what is important, but can wait until later, they are
   a. procrastinating.
   b. hustling.
   c. prioritizing.
   d. ranking.

3. Someone who properly manages their schedule is practicing good
   a. critical thinking.
   b. time management.
   c. note taking.
   d. information literacy.

4. According to the textbook, what is another word for a short-term or long-term achievement that is clearly defined and measurable?
   a. Goal
   b. Hope
   c. Bonus
   d. Endpoint

5. What is the term for seeking solutions to a problem without evaluating the practicality of the idea?
   a. Rallying
   b. Brainstorming
   c. Pitching
   d. Rationalizing

6. The process of _____ includes creativity, making decisions, solving problems, learning new information and reasoning.
   a. brainstorming
   b. critical thinking
   c. prioritizing
   d. time management

7. What is *selective writing*?
   a. Choosing what to listen to
   b. Choosing which notes to write down
   c. Deciding how long to take notes
   d. Choosing what note format to use

8. The Cornell system of note-taking involves drawing a margin line 2.5 inches from the left side and another line about 2 inches from the bottom. The center is for notes during class. What goes in the bottom space?
   a. Questions
   b. Keywords
   c. Summaries
   d. Dates and times

9. One method of reducing test anxiety is by overexposing oneself to the fear with a technique called
   a. desensitization.
   b. visualization.
   c. realization.
   d. self-motivation.

119

10. Information literacy helps people _____ outdated or misinformation.
    a. absorb
    b. recognize
    c. convert
    d. ingest
11. What is the term for a computer program that locates information based on the keywords that are input?
    a. Search engine
    b. Virtual private network
    c. Web Retriever
    d. Software engine
12. Which three letters are the suffix of a government agency website address, such as the FDA or USDA?
    a. .gvt
    b. .gov
    c. .com
    d. .gvn
13. Which of these is an example of computer hardware?
    a. Windows operating system
    b. Electronic Health Record (EHR) program
    c. RAM memory chip
    d. Search engine
14. A data storage server that exists in a remote location and accessed through an Internet connection is called
    a. network bin.
    b. shared space.
    c. cloud computing.
    d. remote airspace.
15. Mr Murray is diabetic and has a continuous glucose monitoring device that allows his blood sugar readings to be sent directly to his provider from his home. This is known as
    a. remote patient monitoring.
    b. rapid test transfer.
    c. off-site patient supervision.
    d. removed patient logging.
16. What is the name for the organizational structure that refers to a chain of command with everyone reporting to a supervisor above them, except for the individual at the top – such as the owner or president?
    a. Team-based
    b. Decentralized
    c. Hierarchical
    d. Divisional

ORGANIZATIONAL AND THINKING SKILLS

Concept Applications

In your own words, complete the chart below. Examples can be from your life as a student or what you might anticipate as a healthcare professional. The first row is completed as an example.

Skill	Definition	Example	Significance
Organization	The process of arranging of items, thinking, and actions in an orderly, efficient manner	Storing your paper, pens, and highlighters in the same spots on your desk all the time	Organization improves efficiency and the ability to complete tasks and achieve goals
Prioritizing			
Time management			
Problem solving			
Critical thinking			

Time Management

Use the following chart to record the time you usually spend each day on the listed activities of daily living. Convert these estimated times to weekly percentages, and draw a pie chart in the circle provided. Each week has 10,080 minutes.

Activity	Time in Minutes
Sleeping	
Eating	
Dressing/undressing	
Exercising	
Reading/study	
School/work	
Leisure activity	
Shopping/errands	
Other:	
Other:	

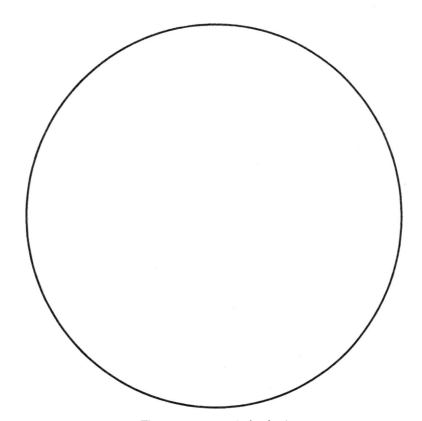

Time management pie chart.

Questions

1. On which activity do you spend the most time?

_____

_____

_____

2. On which activity do you spend more time than you would prefer?

_____

_____

_____

3. On which activity do you spend less time than you would prefer?

_____

_____

_____

4. Can you make any changes in your daily activities that would allow you to spend more time on the activities you prefer?

_____

_____

Goal Setting Checklist

Identify three areas of your personal life or habits that you would like to improve. Examples might be healthy eating, managing finances, keeping your home tidy, or staying on top of your work. Chart in the spaces provided your effort to improve over the next 4 weeks.

GOAL #1: _____

Date	Goal Progress Report
1-week evaluation	
2-week evaluation	
3-week evaluation	
4-week evaluation	

GOAL #2: _____

Date	Goal Progress Report
1-week evaluation	
2-week evaluation	
3-week evaluation	
4-week evaluation	

GOAL #3: _____

Date	Goal Progress Report
1-week evaluation	
2-week evaluation	
3-week evaluation	
4-week evaluation	

Problem-Solving Models

Use these sample story to complete the problem-solving model in the space provided.

Problem 1: You receive your first test back in chemistry class. The grade is a D. You had taken notes during the class lectures, skimmed the chapter, and looked over your notes the night before the test. You had done most of the homework assignments and earned a C grade on them. You know that a grade of D in chemistry could prevent you from going on to an advanced program or college. You want to improve your grade.

Step 1: Recognize that a problem exists. What is the problem?	
Step 2: Clarify the issue. List who is involved and where, when, and how the problem occurred. What other factors affect it?	
Step 3: Identify alternative methods for resolving the problem.	
Step 4: Choose the best method for resolving the problem and implement it. (You may use your imagination to finish the problem.)	
Step 5: Evaluate the results of the method chosen. (You may use your imagination to finish the problem.)	

NOTE-TAKING SKILLS

Practicing the Cornell System

The Cornell system is a method for laying out, editing, and studying from your notes. A key feature of the system is leaving plenty of blank space on each page, so you can add information when you review and edit your notes. On each page, draw a line about 2½ inches from the left side. Then draw a line about 2 inches from the bottom. The large space in the center is for writing your notes during class. You can use the left side after class to write key words, headings, questions, and other notes. The bottom space is for writing short summaries. You can find templates of Cornell notes outlines online. Use the Cornell system to take notes during one class period. Answer the following questions about your experience using this system.

1. How would you describe your experience using the Cornell system of notetaking?

_____

_____

_____

_____

_____

_____

_____

2. What advantages did you notice with the Cornell system? Disadvantages?

_____

_____

_____

_____

_____

3. Did summarizing the notes at the bottom of the page help you understand the material better? Why or why not?

_____

_____

_____

_____

_____

_____

4. Will you use this system again? Why or why not?

_____

_____

_____

_____

_____

_____

TEST TAKING

Practice Tests

One of the best ways to prepare for classroom tests is to create practice questions and quizzes from your notes. Create a practice quiz from your notes for this class. Construct questions in the formats that are typically included on your tests (i.e., multiple choice, short answer, fill-in-the-blank, etc.). Build a separate answer key. Exchange practice quizzes with one or more classmates. Complete the quiz(zes), then return them to the creator(s) for "grading." Review the results. Ask your classmates why they chose to include the material they did on their practice quizzes, and explain your choices as well.

Test Anxiety

Most people are a little nervous before a test. For some, though, the feelings of apprehension and self-doubt can be overwhelming. The textbook describes strategies for managing and improving test anxiety. There are some exercises you can try to help reduce tension. Practice in advance of test day so you are familiar with the method that works best for you.

Breathing Exercise

1. Breathe in gently through your nose, bringing your breath far down into your lungs and expanding your abdomen.
2. Breathe out slowly through your mouth, with your lips slightly pursed and your jaw relaxed.
3. Continue this cycle for 3–5 minutes.

124

Contracting and Releasing Exercise

1. Sit with your feet flat on the floor.
2. Grab under the chair with your hands. Push your feet into the floor and pull the bottom of the chair up with your hands at the same time.
3. Hold for 5 seconds.
4. Release and relax for 5–10 seconds.
5. Repeat the entire process 2–3 times.

Write a paragraph describing your experience with the activity.

_____

_____

_____

_____

_____

INFORMATION LITERACY

Steps for Information Literacy

Using the steps in Box 16-9 of the textbook, choose an acute or chronic health problem you or someone you knows has, or one you are interested in learning more about. Some suggestions include Lyme disease, sleep apnea, age-related macular degeneration, fibromyalgia, lupus, irritable bowel syndrome, Stevens-Johnson syndrome, or leukoplakia.

Step	Your Problem/Actions Taken
Recognize the problem. Create questions. What do you want to know?	
Make a plan for finding information and solutions. How will you find information?	
Formulate hypotheses and make predictions. What do you think you will find?	
Find information and data from books and the Internet. List the sources you used here.	
Evaluate the credibility of the sources.	
Organize and synthesize all gathered information.	
Make conclusions and process understanding.	

125

Internet

The Internet provides a wealth of content. Facts, opinions, sales pitches, entertainment, and a vast array of other material is available with a few taps on a keyboard.

Find an example of each type of information below on the Internet, and indicate its website address. Briefly explain how you determined the category of each type of content.

1. Factual health data:_____

_____

_____

_____

2. Sales of a service (in a format that is not a direct sales advertisement/pitch):

_____

_____

_____

_____

3. Opinion:_____

_____

_____

_____

_____

Computer Literacy

For each choice below, indicate whether it is hardware (H), software (S), or a storage medium (M).

1. ____ Microsoft Windows
2. ____ Mouse
3. ____ EHR system
4. ____ RAM
5. ____ Blank DVD
6. ____ Server
7. ____ E-mail program
8. ____ Thumb USB drive
9. ____ Keyboard
10. ____ Operating system

Cloud Computing

In your own words, explain the concept of cloud computing. Why are the advantages of using this technology?

_____

_____

_____

_____

_____

_____

LEADERSHIP AND ORGANIZATIONAL DEVELOPMENT

Organizational Framework

Organizational development is defined as an effort or process to increase an organization's effectiveness, with the goal of increasing productivity, quality, and worker satisfaction. Organizations are structured in many different ways. Four common organizational structures are hierarchical, functional, divisional, and team. Research two of the four, then answer these questions.

1. Which two structures did you choose?

_____

2. What were the major differences between them?

_____

_____

_____

_____

_____

_____

3. Which do you think would work better? Why?

_____

_____

_____

_____

_____

_____

4. Which structure do you think you'd prefer to work within? Why?

_____

_____

_____

_____

_____

_____

Leadership

You have undoubtedly encountered many leaders in your life, from parents to teachers to the friend who seems to get everyone together. Think of a leader you admire and respect, whether it is someone you know personally or someone you are familiar with from media, then answer these questions based on that person.

1. What characteristics from Box 16-13 in the textbook does the leader you have in mind possess? Give examples of behavior that supports your assertions.

_____

_____

_____

_____

_____

_____

2. What do you admire most about this leader? Why?

_____

_____

_____

_____

_____

_____

3. What leadership qualities do you see in yourself? Explain your answer.

_____

_____

_____

_____

_____

_____

4. What is a leadership quality that you would like to develop within yourself? What are some steps you can take to do that?

_____

_____

_____

_____

_____

_____

17 Physicians and Clinical Support Professionals

CAREERS

Careers, Duties, and Credentials

Using the chapter and other sources, fill in the missing information.

Career Title	Education	Description of Job Duties	Licensure	Credentials
Physician				
Physician assistant				
Medical assistant				CCMA, CMA, CMAA, NCMA, NRCMA

Education Costs and Earnings Potential

Using the Internet, research the educational cost of one physician or clinical support career and the salary that might be earned in the local area. Use the information to complete the table.

Career	Institution for Education	Cost of Education	Potential Earnings

Skills and Qualities

Choose a career discussed in the chapter. List three personal qualities and skills that you think are important for the job and the reason(s) why.

1. _____

2. _____

3. _____

KNOWLEDGE CHECK

Multiple Choice

1. Which is function exclusively the responsibility of the physician?
   a. Patient education
   b. Scheduling patients
   c. Developing the plan of care
   d. Administering medications
2. Which of these is **not** considered a healthcare provider?
   a. Physician assistant
   b. Medical doctor
   c. Dentist
   d. Medical assistant

3. What is the meaning of the term biomechanics?
   a. A set of body measurement tools
   b. A specific calculation involving the patient's height and weight
   c. A visual examination of the patient
   d. The science of moving or manipulation of muscles and bones
4. What is the term for specialized medical training a physician receives?
   a. Scope of practice
   b. Residency
   c. Rounds
   d. Doctorate
5. How long is the *entire* educational experience to become a board-certified specialized surgeon, starting after high school?
   a. 4–6 years
   b. 8 years
   c. 11 years or more
   d. 12 years + residency
6. The position of physician assistant grew out of the need for
   a. less expensive care.
   b. more primary care physicians.
   c. insurance compliance.
   d. more nurses.
7. The HITECH Act of 2008 led many employers to require _____ of medical assistants.
   a. certification or registration
   b. photo identification
   c. background checks
   d. drug testing
8. Clinical medical assistants (CMAs) must earn a certificate or diploma, which can take _____ to complete. They can also complete their education by getting an associate degree, which takes 2 years to complete.
   a. 8 years
   b. 3 months
   c. 3–6 years
   d. 18 months
9. Which term means the process of gathering patient health history, nature of current complaint, and reviewing medical record.
   a. Patient diagnosis
   b. Patient intervention
   c. Patient orientation
   d. Patient interview
10. The inpatient nurse is performing a patient interview on a patient. Which area is not part of the traditional patient interview?
    a. Chief complaint
    b. Social history
    c. Review of test results
    d. Review of systems (ROS)
11. What is the term for a more complete, expansive description of the chief complaint?
    a. History of present illness (HPI)
    b. Diagnosis
    c. Review of systems (ROS)
    d. Vital signs
12. During the patient interview, the patient shares that they "probably drink too much." Which area of the patient interview does this statement fall under?
    a. Review of systems (ROS)
    b. Social history
    c. Chief complain
    d. Family history

13. The final stage of the patient interview is
    a. diagnosis.
    b. review of systems.
    c. current medical history.
    d. chief complaint.
14. Which of these is not a method for measuring a patient's temperature?
    a. Axillary
    b. Oral
    c. Antecubital
    d. Rectal
15. Which piece of equipment measures blood pressure?
    a. Otoscope
    b. Thermometer
    c. Sphygmomanometer
    d. Stethoscope

True/False

Read the following statements and write "T" for true or "F" for false in the blanks provided. If a statement is false, correct the statement to make it true.

1. _____ In the training of a physician, a residency may be followed by a fellowship.
2. _____ A surgeon usually also practices family medicine or internal medicine, referring patients to specialists as needed.
3. _____ A physician assistant can do many of the same things that a physician can do, including writing prescriptions.
4. _____ The education required for a physician assistant is just about the same as that of a MD or DO, though the exams are different.
5. _____ A healthcare professional's scope of practice consists of the activities they are deemed competent to perform.
6. _____ An experienced physician may be able to make a diagnosis based only on patient medical history.
7. _____ Signs are subjective, meaning they vary from case to case, whereas symptoms are objective and observable by others.
8. _____ Basic information that should be obtained for most chief complaints includes past medical history, social history, and family history.
9. _____ Blood pressure consists of two values: systolic, which is the maximum pressure at which the pulse can be heard, and diastolic, the minimum pressure at which the pulse can be heard.
10. _____ A normal adult pulse rate is between 100 and 160 beats per minute (BPM).
11. _____ The tip of the stem of the rectal thermometer is red, and that of the oral thermometer is blue or silver for easy identification.

Matching

Match the numbered term below with the best definition.

Terms	Definition
1. _____ Inspection	a. Striking the body to assess the sound made
2. _____ Palpation	b. Examination technique of listening to the body's sounds
3. _____ Anthropometric measurements	c. Visual examination of the patient
4. _____ Percussion	d. Measurements of the size, shape, and composition of the human body
5. _____ Auscultation	e. The inspiration and expiration of a breath
6. _____ Vital signs	f. Examination technique of feeling for size, texture, consistency with hands
7. _____ Respiration	g. Collection of measurements taken to assess bodily function and detect changes in condition

Chapter **17** **Physicians and Clinical Support Professionals**

CONTENT INSTRUCTION

The Patient Interview

Review the guidelines for conducting the patient interview in Box 17-3. For each of the scenarios below, identify what was done incorrectly, and then suggest a correction.

1. The healthcare provider enters the room and immediately says to the patient, "The receptionist said you were having nausea. How long has that been going on?"
2. Important test results should be coming in any moment. The healthcare provider glances at her phone a few times while the patient is sharing his chief complaint to see if the results are available.
3. The healthcare provider asks the patient, "Are you experiencing chest pain, tingling, or muscle weakness?"
4. The patient says she is experiencing frequent headaches. The healthcare provider says, "That's every day, right?"

SIGNS VS SYMPTOMS

Indicate whether each description is a sign or a symptom.

1. Chest pain   _____
2. 101.2°F   _____
3. Swollen thumb   _____
4. Ringing in ears   _____
5. Nausea   _____
6. Rash on foot   _____
7. Leg numbness   _____
8. Laceration on palm   _____
9. Heart rate of 66 bpm   _____
10. 124/80 blood pressure   _____
11. Fatigue   _____

PAST MEDICAL HISTORY

For your own information, compile your past medical history. Include the components listed in Box 17-4 in the textbook. This is for your own use. You will not include it in the workbook or share it with the instructor or the class.

PERFORMANCE APPLICATION

Taking a Blood Pressure Reading

Read all of the instructions before beginning this activity. Laboratory activities should be completed under the supervision of a qualified professional only.

Equipment and Supplies

Stethoscope, sphygmomanometer, alcohol pad, pen, and paper

Directions

1. Maintain medical asepsis by using the guidelines provided in the Standard and Transmission-Based Precautions, including good handwashing technique and use of gloves as needed.
2. Gather all necessary equipment, including a stethoscope, sphygmomanometer, alcohol pad, pen, and paper.
3. Identify the patient and explain the procedure. Identification of the correct patient and explanation of the procedure prevents errors and misunderstanding.
4. Position the patient in either a sitting or lying position with the upper arm exposed and supported above the level of the heart. Clothing must allow exposure of the upper arm completely without binding. Privacy should be provided if necessary. Either arm may be used, but arms with injuries, IV lines, or other treatments should be avoided, because the procedure may cause injury or pain, or the reading may be inaccurate.
5. Wrap the cuff of the sphygmomanometer around the arm 1 inch above the bend of the elbow (antecubital space) to allow room for the flat placement of the stethoscope. The cuff should be tight enough that two fingers may be placed under the edge comfortably. If the cuff is too tight or too loose, the reading will be inaccurate.

6. While palpating the radial artery, tighten the thumbscrew of the sphygmomanometer, and inflate until the pulse disappears. This reading is an approximate systolic pressure.

7. Deflate the cuff completely and allow the arm to rest for 30 seconds.

8. Clean the earplugs of the stethoscope with alcohol and place them into the ears with the opening pointing toward the nose.

9. Locate the brachial pulse with the tips of two fingers and place the flat part (diaphragm) of the stethoscope on the location of the pulse. Placement over the brachial artery allows the pulse to be heard more easily (audible) when the cuff is inflated.

10. Tighten the thumbscrew valve by turning it clockwise, and inflate the cuff to 20–30 mm Hg above the approximate systolic value.

11. Deflate the cuff, slowly noting the location on the scale at which the first (systolic) and last (diastolic) pulse are heard. The last distinct beat is considered to be the diastolic pulse. Soft muffled or thumping sounds are not counted.

12. Deflate the cuff completely after the BP is assessed and remove the cuff from the arm. The blood pressure can be reassessed using the same arm a second time. If a third reading is necessary, the cuff should be removed briefly between readings or moved to the other arm because tightening the cuff repeatedly may change the pressure.

13. Record the results. Report any unusual findings to the supervisor immediately. An elevated or low blood pressure may signal an emergency situation.

14. Store equipment in the designated area and discard the alcohol pad in an appropriate container.

Measurements

Time of Reading	Systolic	Diastolic

Taking an Infrared Temperature

Read all of the instructions before beginning this activity. Laboratory activities should be completed under the supervision of a qualified professional only.

Equipment and Supplies

Thermal thermometer, alcohol, swab, pen, and paper

Directions

1. Maintain medical asepsis by using the guidelines provided in the Standard and Transmission-Based Precautions, including good handwashing technique and use of gloves as needed.

2. Gather all necessary equipment and supplies, including a thermal thermometer, alcohol swab, pen, and paper.

3. Press the power button to activate the thermometer.

4. Check that the thermometer is set for the preferred mode (Fahrenheit or Celsius).

5. Press and hold "scan" until the image "00" appears on the screen.

6. Hold the thermometer about 2–3 inches away from and in the middle of the forehead.

7. While holding the "scan" button, move the thermometer toward and away from the forehead until it beeps continuously and the light flashes.

8. When the beeping is continuous, release the "scan" button. The thermometer will beep once and show the temperature.

9. The thermometer will automatically shut off.

10. Use an alcohol swab to clean the thermometer lens. Store it in the designated area.

11. Discard the alcohol swab or pledget in an appropriate container. Maintain medical asepsis by washing your hands for a minimum of 20 seconds.

Measurements

Time of Reading	Temperature (Fahrenheit)	Temperature (Celsius)

133

Copyright © 2023 Elsevier, Inc. All rights reserved.

Chapter **17** **Physicians and Clinical Support Professionals**

Medical Doctors and Doctors of Osteopathic Medicine

Medical doctors (MDs) and doctors of osteopathy (DOs) both complete bachelor's degrees, medical school, and residencies. Differences do exist between them. In addition to the 200 hours of training in manipulation techniques that candidates for the DO degree complete, practitioners of osteopathy have a different orientation than traditional allopathically trained medical doctors. The philosophy of osteopathic medicine is based on the belief that the human body is an integrated organism with a natural ability to resist disease and heal itself. (*Answers will vary.*)

1. How do you think this philosophy differs from that of allopathic medicine?

_____

_____

_____

_____

_____

_____

_____

2. Given the choice, would you have a preference for your own primary care provider? Why or why not?

_____

_____

_____

_____

_____

_____

Social History

Review Box 17-5, Information Included in a Social History. Some of the questions posed during the taking of a social history are very personal. It might be uncomfortable or embarrassing to answer them honestly, especially if you have not yet developed a good relationship with the healthcare provider who's asking them.

1. Why do you think this information is considered relevant to your health history?

_____

_____

_____

_____

_____

_____

2. Do you think it is important to answer questions about social history honestly? Why or why not?

_____

_____

_____

_____

_____

_____

_____

3. What might be some consequences of refusing to provide social history information, or providing false information?

_____

_____

_____

_____

_____

_____

_____

_____

4. Why is it important that a healthcare provider keep patient information confidential?

_____

_____

_____

_____

_____

_____

_____

_____

_____

135

18 Nursing Professionals

Careers, Duties, and Credentials

Using the chapter and other sources, fill in the missing information.

Career Title	Education	Description of Job Duties	Licensure	Credentials
				LPN or LVN via NCLEX-PN
Registered nurse				*RN via NCLEX-RN*
	State-approved certification program			CNA via certification exam
Advanced practice registered nurse				Specialty certifications available

Education Costs and Earnings Potential

Using the Internet, research the educational cost of one nursing career and the salary that might be earned in the local area. Use the information to complete the table.

Career	Institution for Education	Cost of Education	Potential Earnings

Skills and Qualities

Choose a career discussed in the chapter. List three personal qualities and skills that you think are important for the job and the reason(s) why.

1. _____

_____

_____

2. _____

_____

_____

3. _____

_____

_____

Interviewing a Nurse

The nursing profession comprises the largest healthcare profession, with more than 3.5 million working in a wide range of healthcare settings and fields. If you know a nurse, ask if he or she would be willing to talk to you about his or her profession. Use the questions below to guide the conversation. If you do not know a nurse, visit one of the professional association websites listed in the textbook, and think of several possible answers for a typical healthcare professional in one of the nursing categories discussed in this chapter.

1. What setting do you work in?

_____

_____

2. What are your typical responsibilities?

_____

_____

_____

_____

_____

3. What path did you take to get to this point in your career?

_____

_____

_____

_____

4. What is the most rewarding part of your job?

_____

_____

_____

_____

5. What is the most challenging part of your job?

_____

_____

_____

_____

KNOWLEDGE CHECK

Multiple Choice

Circle the one correct answer to each of the following questions.

1. Which of these levels of nursing requires the least amount of training and education?
   a. RN
   b. APRN
   c. Nurse practitioner
   d. LPN

2. Which type of nurse might supervise nursing students?
   a. LPN
   b. LVM
   c. RN
   d. Nursing assistant

3. BSN nursing students' education includes leadership and management, whereas ADN and diploma nursing students learn mostly _____ skills.
   a. interpersonal
   b. clinical
   c. research
   d. specialty

4. In 2019, the average annual pay for a registered nurse (RN) fell within which range?
   a. $20,000–$30,000
   b. $35,000–$40,000
   c. $40,000–$50,000
   d. $70,000–$80,000

5. A registered nurse student must graduate from school and pass which exam?
   a. NCLEX-CME
   b. NCLEX-PN
   c. NCLEX-RN
   d. NCLEX-BSN

6. What is the current trend in nursing education?
   a. To encourage more nurses to obtain a BSN
   b. To encourage more nurses to obtain a master's degree
   c. To create more diploma programs
   d. To train more LPNs

7. What is the purpose of a nurse bridging program?
   a. To get nurses acquainted with co-workers
   b. To allow nurses to cross over into other areas of medicine
   c. To support nurses with degrees who wish to move to a higher academic nursing level
   d. To provide financial assistance while the student is in early stages of nursing school

8. Which nursing position is a level above registered nurse (RN)?
   a. CNA
   b. LPN
   c. LVN
   d. APRN

9. The average annual salary of a nurse practitioner in the U.S. in 2019 falls between which range?
   a. $65,000 and $75,000
   b. $85,000 and $95,000
   c. $36,000 and $45,000
   d. $115,000 and $125,000

10. Which is an instrumental activity of daily living (IADL)?
    a. Grooming
    b. Toileting
    c. Preparing food
    d. Eating food

11. Nursing assistants (NAs) work under the supervision of a RN or LPN and mainly provide _____ to patients.
    a. patient education
    b. medications
    c. diagnoses
    d. basic and personal care

12. The average annual pay for a nursing assistant in the U.S. in 2019 was between
    a. $50,000 and $65,000
    b. $75,000 and $85,000
    c. $26,000 and $35,000
    d. $130,000 and $145,000

13. What does the "A" stand for in the acronym "ADPIE," which explains the five steps in the nursing process?
    a. Assessment
    b. Activity
    c. Attention
    d. Agreement

14. Severe diarrhea could lead to
    a. dehydration.
    b. anorexia nervosa.
    c. pneumonia.
    d. blindness.

15. Which form of fluid loss cannot be measured?
    a. Emesis
    b. Urine
    c. Liquid stool
    d. Perspiration

16. In addition to wearing PPE, handwashing is one of the best ways to prevent spread of pathogens. How long should you wash your hands?
    a. no more than 10 seconds
    b. no more than 1 minute
    c. at least 2 minutes
    d. at least 20 seconds

17. The Centers for Disease Control and Prevention (CDC) recommends a set of safety measures including handwashing, using protective barriers and PPE. What is this set of measures called?
    a. Safety Precautions
    b. Safety Preparations
    c. Standard Precautions
    d. Standard Preparations

18. Mrs Robinson has spent 3 months in a long-term care facility. The staff did not reposition her frequently enough and now she has skin breakdown where she laid. What is another term for this type of injury?
    a. Dermatitis
    b. Blood clot
    c. Scabies
    d. Decubitus ulcer

True or False

Read the following statements and write "T" for true or "F" for false in the blanks provided. If a statement is false, correct the statement to make it true.

_____ 1. Registered nurses may practice under the supervision of a physician, or independently in areas such as women's health.

_____ 2. Most states require nursing assistants to become certified.

_____ 3. Nursing assistants must complete a 1- or 2-year training program.

_____ 4. Oral intake is considered anything that is liquid at room temperature and taken by mouth.

_____ 5. Range-of-motion exercises may be ordered for patients who are immobile, and should be performed at least once every 24 hours.

_____ 6. One of the most important safety practices used by nursing staff is checking the identification of the patient before administering medications.

_____ 7. Transmission-based precautions are observed when standard precautions are not necessary.

_____ 8. When assisting a patient with eating, it is important to refrain from talking.

_____ 9. When making a bed, linens will be used in this order: pillowcases, bottom sheet, mattress pad, draw sheet, top sheet, blanket, and bedspread.

_____ 10. It is not possible to make a bed while it is occupied by the patient.

Matching

Match the body position with its application.

Position	Application
_____ 1. Supine	a. Raises only the legs, may be used to treat conditions of lowered blood pressure such as shock
_____ 2. Prone	b. Taking a rectal temperature or administering enemas
_____ 3. Semi-Fowlers	c. May be used for comfort or to decrease pressure on the abdominal organs
_____ 4. Left Sims'	d. Ease respiratory distress
_____ 5. Orthopneic	e. Comfort or sleep
_____ 6. Trendelenberg	f. Treatments to the back

CONTENT INSTRUCTION

Nursing Process

Registered and advanced practice nurses may follow a series of steps with the acronym ADPIE: Assessment, Diagnosis, Planning, Implementation, and Evaluation (see Box 18-6). Determine which step each of these actions is considered.

Action	ADPIE Step
Perform massage on patient	
Take initial vital signs and patient history, review diagnostic and lab reports	
Review patient vital signs and labs, speak with patient about their level of distress or comfort after treatment	
Determine patient has a risk for falling	
Determine actions that would help patient breathe more easily and loosen congestion	

Maintaining the Unit

Skills List 18-3 details steps to maintain the unit. Provide a rationale for each.

Step	Example or Rationale
Maintain medical asepsis by using the guidelines provided in the Standard and Transmission-based Precautions, including good handwashing technique and use of gloves as needed.	
Change the sheets daily and when soiled. Remove soiled linens from the room frequently.	
Replace equipment, supplies, and the patient's possessions to the designated location after each use.	
Throw trash in the appropriate location and empty frequently.	
Supply the patient with fresh water once a shift and as needed.	
Clean surfaces of tables regularly and as soiled.	
Always keep the call bell within reach of the patient.	

Fill in the Blank

Fill in each of the spaces provided with the missing word or words that complete the sentence.

1. _____ are different areas of the hospital not considered departments which provide specialized patient care and special care wards.

2. Data for the nursing assessment step of ADPIE is gathered by interviewing the patient, physical _____ and observation.

3. The clinical term for vomit is _____.

4. When performing range-of-motion exercises, the patient should be positioned comfortably in the _____ position.

5. Sheets that are free of wrinkles are more comfortable and help prevent the formation of _____.

6. The nursing _____ manual is one resource used to guide staff members regarding security practices.

7. Compared to oral consumption, intravenous (IV) fluids and tube feeding are considered more invasive methods of providing _____.

8. The "I" in ADPIE stands for _____ or _____.

9. Hospital beds are often made with _____ corners, a bed-making technique that creates a sharp, smooth corner. (*mitered*)

10. The nursing process ADPIE is a _____ -oriented framework for meeting the patient's needs.

PERFORMANCE APPLICATION

Measuring Oral Intake

Monitoring fluid intake and output is an important responsibility of nursing staff. Practice monitoring your own fluid intake over the course of 24 hours. Remember that anything that is liquid at room temperature and consumed by mouth is considered a fluid.

Time of Day	Liquid Substance	Amount

Reading an EHR

Figure 18-1 is a graphic tab of an electronic health record (EHR) showing the vital signs for Mrs Martha Jewel during a 5-day stay in the hospital. Use the information in the figure to answer the following questions.

1. Why was Mrs Jewel admitted to the hospital?

_____

_____

_____

2. When did Mrs Jewel run a fever during her stay?

_____

_____

3. When was the highest blood pressure reading taken during Mrs Jewel's stay?

_____

_____

_____

4. On which postoperative day, did Mrs Jewel leave the hospital?

_____

_____

5. When were the vital signs for Mrs Jewel omitted during her stay?

_____

_____

6. What is the name of Mrs Jewel's doctor?

_____

_____

_____

CRITICAL THINKING

Diploma vs Associate vs Bachelor's Registered Nurse

For several decades, state and federal governments, nursing associations, and healthcare systems have been pushing to make BSN qualifications mandatory for all nurses. What are pros and cons of this movement?

_____

_____

_____

_____

_____

_____

_____

_____

Calm, Caring, and Professional

The textbook states, "The manner and method in which the health professional provides personal care often determines the patient's reaction to having someone assist with these activities or treatments." What are some of the things that would be important to you if you were receiving personal care from a healthcare professional? What are some behaviors or attitudes that you would find difficult or offensive?

_____

_____

_____

_____

_____

_____

_____

143

Nursing Shortage

The demand for nurses has intensified in the United States and is expected to continue to do so. Reasons for this include an aging and longer-lived population, the retirement of older nurses, and more access to healthcare via the Affordable Care Act of 2010. Nursing schools lack the faculty, facilities, and training sites to meet the growing demand. What are three strategies you think might help meet the demand for working nurses?

_____

_____

_____

_____

_____

_____

_____

_____

_____

19 Pharmacists and Pharmacy Support Staff

Careers, Duties, and Credentials

Using the chapter and other sources, fill in the missing information.

CAREER TITLE	EDUCATION	DESCRIPTION OF JOB DUTIES	LICENSURE	CREDENTIALS
				CPhT via the PTCB or NHA
Pharmacy assistant				
	Postgraduate professional degree (PharmD)			

Education Costs and Earnings Potential

Using the Internet, research the educational cost of one of the pharmacy-related careers discussed in this chapter, and the salary that might be earned in the local area. Use the information to complete the table.

CAREER	INSTITUTION FOR EDUCATION	COST OF EDUCATION	POTENTIAL EARNINGS

Skills and Qualities

Choose a career discussed in the chapter. List three personal qualities and skills that you think are important for the job and the reason(s) why.

1. _____

2. _____

3. _____

KNOWLEDGE CHECK

Multiple Choice

Instructions: Circle the one correct answer to each of the following questions.

1. What is the name for a company that contracts with an employer, health insurer, or government payer to negotiate drug prices and offer prescription needs to beneficiaries?
   a. Primary provider
   b. Pharmacy benefit manager
   c. Covered entity
   d. Retail pharmacist

2. What is the term for the list of drugs available to a health insurance enrollee?
   a. ExpressScripts
   b. Formulary
   c. Prescription instructions
   d. Standing order

3. A *practicing pharmacist* has a _____, while a *professional pharmacist* has a _____.
   a. high school education or equivalent; 2-year associate degree
   b. 2-year associate degree; 4-year bachelor's degree
   c. 5-year PharmB; 6-year PharmD
   d. 6-year PharmD; 5-year PharmB

4. Some pharmacy schools accept students directly after high school graduation and are referred to as _____ programs.
   a. HS+6
   b. PharmD-6
   c. 0–6
   d. 18+

5. After completing the PharmD program, a prospective pharmacist must pass which exam(s)?
   a. North American Pharmacist Licensure exam (NAPLEX)
   b. Multistate Pharmacy Jurisprudence exam (MPJE)
   c. The American Council for Pharmacy Education exam (ACPEX) *and* the Multistate Pharmacy Jurisprudence exam
   d. The North American Pharmacist Licensure exam (NAPLEX) *and* the Multistate Pharmacy Jurisprudence exam (MPJE)

6. The pharmacy assistant is a(n) _____ staff member.
   a. clinical
   b. entry-level
   c. medical
   d. highly trained

7. Another term for a community pharmacy is a _____ pharmacy.
   a. wholesale
   b. mail order
   c. market
   d. retail

8. The pharmacist technician in a hospital might fill over 1000 individual prescriptions, which are picked up by the _____ and administered to the patient.
   a. toxicologist
   b. patient or caregiver
   c. attending physician
   d. nurse

9. Polypharmacy is when
   a. a patient visits more than one pharmacy.
   b. a retail store contains an in-house pharmacy along with vitamins and minerals.
   c. a pharmacy takes many different types of insurance.
   d. a patient takes multiple medications at the same time.

10. Which of these tasks might the pharmacy technician or pharmacist do, but not a pharmacy assistant?
    a. Answer phones
    b. Monitor inventory
    c. Perform dosage calculations
    d. Greet patients

11. Which controlled substance class, or schedule, has the highest potential for abuse and addiction?
    a. Schedule V
    b. Schedule I
    c. Schedule VII
    d. Schedule Zero
12. The generic name for a medication is created by the
    a. FDA.
    b. drug company.
    c. pharmacy.
    d. DEA.
13. Generic medications generally cost how much less than their brand-name equivalent?
    a. 10%
    b. 25%
    c. 50%
    d. 85%
14. Which abbreviation would appear on a prescription, if not e-prescribed, to indicate the patient should take the medication at bedtime.
    a. p.r.n.
    b. h.s.
    c. q.d.
    d. b.i.d.
15. Inunction is a route of drug administration that involves applying medication
    a. into a body orifice.
    b. inside the cheek.
    c. topically to the skin.
    d. under the tongue.

True/False

Instructions: Read the following statements and write "T" for true or "F" for false in the blanks provided. If a statement is false, correct the statement to make it true.

_____ 1. A pharmacy technician has the authority to fill prescriptions and a pharmacy assistant cannot.

_____ 2. Pharmacy technicians can earn the CPhT credential if they pass either the PTCE or the ExCPT tests. They do not need to pass both.

_____ 3. While you will find both PharmD, or "professional pharmacists," and BS Pharm, or "practicing pharmacists" working today, the current industry standard is the BS Pharm degree.

_____ 4. E-prescribing can create more confusion in the doctor's office and the pharmacy because of the high possibility of an error versus traditional paper prescriptions.

_____ 5. Pharmacists who work in research and development (R&D) in the pharmaceutical industry are referred to as toxicologists.

_____ 6. Clinical trials conducted in the development of new drugs take 2–4 years, on average, to complete.

_____ 7. It is important to obtain information about medications that a patient stopped taking within the past 30 days.

_____ 8. The three common systems of measurement used to calculate drug dosages are apothecary, parenteral, and metric.

_____ 9. According to the National Center for Health Statistics (NCHS), almost half of adults in the United States take at least one prescription drug.

_____ 10. The inscription on a prescription is the pharmacist's signature.

CONTENT INSTRUCTION

Matching: Drug Classifications According to the Controlled Substances Act of 1970

Match each characteristic, regulation, or drug in column A with the corresponding Drug Schedule number to which it belongs in column B by writing the appropriate numeral in the space provided. (Note that responses may be used more than once.)

Column A	Column B
1. _____ Opium	Schedule I
2. _____ Low potential for abuse	Schedule II
3. _____ Moderate potential for abuse	Schedule III
4. _____ No accepted use in the United States	Schedule IV
5. _____ Oral emergency orders may be given, but physician must supply written prescription within 72 hours	Schedule V
6. _____ Adderall	
7. _____ Valium	
8. _____ May be refilled five times in 6 months with prescription authorization by physician	
9. _____ Lomotil	
10. _____ Accepted medicinal use with specific restrictions	
11. _____ For research use only	
12. _____ PCP	
13. _____ Methadone	
14. _____ High potential for abuse	
15. _____ Potential for high psychological dependence, low physical dependence	
16. _____ Phenobarbital	
17. _____ Limited psychological and physical dependence with use	
18. _____ Buyer must be 18 years of age or older, show ID, and sign for medications	

Fill in the Chart: Common Pharmacology Abbreviations

Using the chapter and other sources, fill in the missing information.

Abbreviation	Meaning
	By mouth, orally
	Dispense as written
d.c.	
	Four times a day
	Drop
Top	
b.s.	
XD	

Abbreviation	Meaning
b.i.d.	
q	
EOD	
	Quantity
q.o.d.	
	As needed
	Take before meals
PA	

Comparing Fluid Measurements

Three systems are currently used to measure fluid volumes: metric, apothecary, and household units. The metric system, developed in France, is used internationally, and is based on the decimal system, using units of 10. The apothecary system was the original system used in the United States by pharmacists. The household system was developed for use with common items found in the home. Study the chart of approximate equivalents to answer the questions.

Metric	Apothecary	Household
1000 mL	32 oz	1 qt
500 mL	16 oz	1 pt
30 mL	1 oz	2 T
4 mL	1 dr	1 tsp
0.06 mL	1 min	1 gt

Key to Symbols
cc=cubic centimeter
mL=milliliter
oz=fluid ounce (℥)
dr=fluid dram (ℨ)
min=fluid minim (♏)
qt=quart
pt=pint
T=tablespoon
tsp=teaspoon
gt=drop

1. How many ounces are equivalent to 60 cc?

   _____

2. How many milliliters are equivalent to 1 teaspoon?

   _____

3. How many cubic centimeters are equivalent to 10 ounces'?

   _____

4. How many liters are equivalent to 1200 cc?

   _____

5. Which system is most easily changed from one unit of measurement to another in the same system?

   _____

Calculating Drug Dosages

Use the table below to calculate the following dosage problems.

Apothecary Units	Metric Units	Household Units
15–16 minims (min)	1 mL (cc)	
1 fluid dram	4 mL (cc)	1 teaspoon or 60 drops (gtt)
	16 mL	1 tablespoon
1 fluid ounce (oz)	30 mL	
1 quart (qt)	1000 mL (1 L)	
1/60 grain (gr)	1 mg	
1 gr	0.065 g	
15 gr	1 g	
2.2 lb	1 kg	
Examples	Because 1 kg = 2.2 lb, change pounds to kilograms by dividing the number of pounds by 2.2.12	
	0 lb/2.2 (lb/kg) = 54.05 kg	
	Because 1 oz = 30 mL, change ounces to milliliters by multiplying the number of ounces by 30.8	
	oz×30 mL/oz = 240 mL	

1. The order is to give the client a medication at the dosage of 10 mL every hour. What would the correct dosage be in teaspoons?

_____

2. The order is to give the client a medication at the dosage of 300 mg. You have tablets that are 500 mg in strength. How many tablets would you need to give the client for a correct dosage?

_____

3. The order is to give the client a medication at the dosage of 15 mg/kg of weight, three times a day. You have a dosage of grains. The client weighs 120 pounds. How much of the medication do you need to have on hand for a 24-hour period?

_____

CRITICAL THINKING

1. An increasing number of states are requiring pharmacy technicians to complete a training program that is accredited by the American Society of Health-System Pharmacists (ASHP). What are some pros and cons of this requirement?

_____

_____

_____

_____

_____

_____

_____

_____

_____

_____

_____

_____

2. In 1971, the U.S. Congress passed the Controlled Substances Act, which established federal drug policy under which the manufacture, importation, possession, use and distribution of certain substances is regulated. As a result of the Act, prescribed medications and controlled substances are classified based on their medical use in treatment and potential for abuse. Do you think the need exists for revisions to the Controlled Substances Act? Why or why not?

_____

_____

_____

_____

_____

_____

_____

_____

_____

_____

_____

_____

151

20 Respiratory Care Professionals

CAREERS

Careers, Duties, and Credentials

Using the chapter and other sources, fill in the missing information.

CAREER TITLE	EDUCATION	DESCRIPTION OF JOB DUTIES	LICENSURE	CREDENTIALS
			Licensed in some states and registered in some others	CPSGT, RPGST, RST
Respiratory therapist			All states except Alaska require licensure	
Respiratory therapy technician			Some states require registration	

Education Costs and Earnings Potential

Using the Internet, research the educational cost of a career in respiratory care and the salary that might be earned in the local area. Use the information to complete the table.

CAREER	INSTITUTION FOR EDUCATION	COST OF EDUCATION	POTENTIAL EARNINGS

Skills and Qualities

Choose a career discussed in the chapter. List three personal qualities and skills that you think are important for the job and the reason(s) why.

1. _____

2. _____

3. _____

Multiple Choice

Circle the one correct answer to each of the following questions.

1. What is the role of a polysomnographic technician?
   a. To evaluate and assess a patient's sleep health
   b. To clean respiratory equipment under the supervision of a respiratory therapist
   c. To manage life support equipment
   d. To read, evaluate, and diagnose chest X-rays

2. A respiratory therapist cares for patients with cardiopulmonary health issues. What is the minimum education needed for this profession?
   a. High-school diploma + 1200 hours internship
   b. Associate degree
   c. Bachelor's degree + 1200 hours internship
   d. Master's degree

3. Which body structures are described by the term *cardiopulmonary*?
   a. Lungs and stomach
   b. Lungs and brain
   c. Brain and heart
   d. Lungs and heart

4. One of the functions of the respiratory system is maintaining the blood's _____ balance.
   a. red blood cell
   b. white blood cell
   c. hormone
   d. electrolyte

5. What is the medical term for the cavity that contains the heart and lungs?
   a. Dorsal
   b. Ventral
   c. Thorax
   d. Ventrical

6. What is the medical term for *normal* breathing?
   a. Eupnea
   b. Apnea
   c. Dyspnea
   d. Orthopnea

7. What is the meaning of the term *dyspnea*?
   a. General difficulty breathing
   b. Trouble breathing, but only lying down
   c. Cessation of breathing
   d. Trouble breathing, but only when lying on one side

8. Ms Rogers was diagnosed with pneumonia and has difficulty breathing, but only when lying on her side. This form of difficult breathing is called
   a. trepopnea.
   b. orthopnea.
   c. apnea.
   d. hypoventilation.

9. Hypoventilation leads to increased _____ levels which makes the blood more acidic, leading to confusion, muscle dysfunction, and irregular heartbeat.
   a. cardon dioxide
   b. oxygen
   c. nitrogen
   d. glucose

10. What is the brand name for the product that can be injected to reverse the effects of anaphylaxis, a severe allergic reaction?
    a. NepStick®
    b. EpiStick®
    c. NephriPen®
    d. EpiPen®
11. Which condition is diagnosed when a person ceases to breathe for lengths of time throughout the night?
    a. Tachypnea
    b. Obstructive sleep apnea
    c. Somnambulism
    d. Chronic hypoxemia
12. *Phlegm* is mucus in the
    a. vagina.
    b. mouth.
    c. lungs.
    d. nose.
13. *Purulent sputum* is a sign of
    a. too much carbon dioxide.
    b. a bacterial infection.
    c. internal bleeding.
    d. a respiratory obstruction.
14. If a patient is suspected to have sleep apnea, a sleep study might be performed which monitors an array of physiological activities as the patient sleeps. This study is called
    a. electrocardiography (EKG).
    b. electroencephalogram (EEG).
    c. electrosomnogram (ESG).
    d. polysomnography (PSG).
15. Which diagnostic tool measures the volume of air the lungs can hold and the speed that a patient can expel it?
    a. Pulse oximeter
    b. Spirometer
    c. Peak flow monitor
    d. Arterial blood gas (ABG) test

True/False
Read the following statements and write "T" for true or "F" for false in the blanks provided. If a statement is false, correct the statement to make it true.

_____ 1. Respiratory therapy assistants administer routine respiratory care under the supervision of an RT or physician.

_____ 2. A respiratory therapist (RT) can practice without an advanced degree as long as they pass the examination and complete an internship under a registered RT.

_____ 3. Cold weather and cockroaches are two possible triggers for patients with asthma.

_____ 4. Exhalation occurs when the diaphragm relaxes, expelling carbon dioxide into the air.

_____ 5. The buildup of excessive moisture impairs breathing in patients with asthma.

_____ 6. The most accurate way to measure a patient's acid-base balance as well as oxygen and carbon dioxide levels is with an arterial blood gas (ABG) test.

_____ 7. Spirometry measures the amount of oxygen in the blood using a clip-like probe.

_____ 8. Tapping the patient to try and identify the abnormal presence of fluid of air is called *palpation*.

_____ 9. The tidal volume is the total amount of air that can be exchanged by an individual.

_____ 10. Disturbances in the body's acid–base balance that indicate a breathing problem are called metabolic acidosis or metabolic alkalosis. Metabolic acidosis results from too much acid being produced or not enough being cleared; it might mean the patient has diabetes, kidney problems, or is severely dehydrated. Metabolic alkalosis can result from prolonged vomiting or hypovolemia (decreased blood volume).

_____ 11. Tachypnea is an abnormally rapid breathing of respiratory rate greater than 20 breaths per minute.

Matching

Match the condition with the description.

1. _____	Chronic obstructive pulmonary disease (COPD)	A. Inflammation and narrowing of the airways
2. _____	Asthma	B. Inflammation of the bronchial tubes
3. _____	Pleurisy	C. Viral infection of the trachea and larynx in children
4. _____	Bronchitis	D. Partially collapsed lung
5. _____	Pulmonary fibrosis	E. Genetic disease in which the body produces a sticky mucus that can clog
6. _____	Croup	F. The blocking of the airway through bronchiolitis
7. _____	Pneumoconiosis	G. Inflammation of the outside lining of the lungs causing pain
8. _____	Atelectasis	H. Lung disease caused by inhaling dust particles
9. _____	Emphysema	I. Damage and scarring of the lungs
10. _____	Cystic fibrosis	J. Irreversible abnormal enlargement and destruction of the alveoli that perform gas exchange

Understanding the Concepts

Visit the American Lung Association website listed under Advocacy and Research Organizations at the end of Chapter 20 in the textbook. Spend a few moments looking at the information categories and topics there.

Choose one of the topics on the website to research (examples include Lung Health & Wellness, How Lungs Work, E-Cigarettes & Vaping, Radon, Particle Pollution, etc.). Create a PowerPoint presentation or a written report about your topic and answer the following questions.

1. Why did you choose this topic to research?

_____

_____

_____

_____

2. What was the most interesting thing you learned in your research?

_____

_____

_____

_____

3. Was there any information in your research that you found personally useful?

_____

_____

_____

_____

_____

4. Which respiratory health professionals, if any, do you think might be involved in this area?

_____

_____

_____

_____

_____

PERFORMANCE INSTRUCTION

Performing a Lung Volume Reading

The volume of air moved into and out of the lung may be used to measure the ability of the body to supply oxygen to the cells. If a wet spirometer is not available for this activity, a large, water-filled jar on which the volume is indicated may be substituted (Figure 20-1). Read all directions before beginning this activity. Laboratory activities should be performed under the supervision of a qualified professional only.

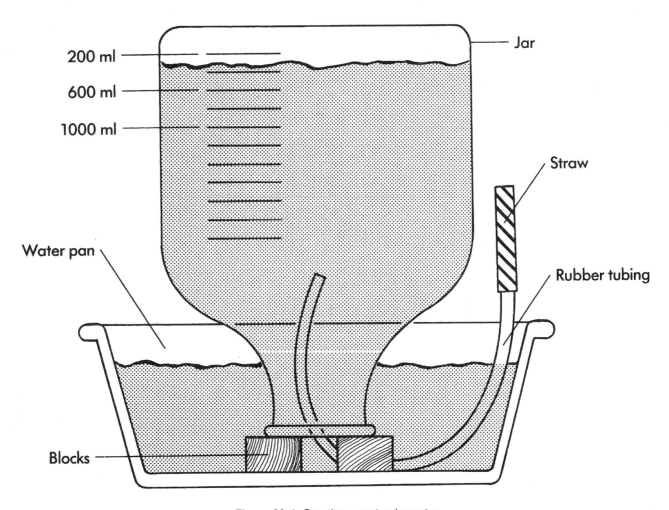

Figure 20-1 Creating a wet spirometer.

Chapter **20 Respiratory Care Professionals**

Equipment and Supplies
Disposable mouthpieces
Wet spirometer or jar apparatus

Directions

1. Work in groups of at least two people.
2. Assemble a wet spirometer for lung volume readings. Read the manufacturer's instructions before beginning. Some wet spirometers require inspiration of air instead of exhalation as later described. Exhalation is used to measure when the jar apparatus is used.
3. Place a disposable mouthpiece in the breathing tube.
4. Do not look at the gauge during breathing trials. Your partner should read all measurements.
5. To measure the tidal volume, breathe at a normal rate for several minutes. When the normal volume of air for one breath is inhaled through the mouth, gently exhale through the mouthpiece. Perform this measurement three times, and compute the average of the resulting volumes.

   Trial 1 _____liters

   Trial 2 _____liters   Average = _____ liters

   Trial 3 _____liters   Tidal Volume

6. To measure your inspiratory reserve, inhale as much air as possible. Breathe the air gently through the mouthpiece until you reach the end of a normal breath. This measurement includes the tidal volume. Perform this measurement three times, and compute the average of the resulting volumes.

   Trial 1 _____liters

   Trial 2 _____liters   Average = _____liters

   Trial 3 _____liters   Inspiratory Reserve + Tidal Volume

   Because the inspiratory reserve that you measured contains the tidal volume, you must subtract the average tidal volume from the measured inspiratory reserve to get the true value of the inspiratory reserve.

   Average = _____ liters

   Total Inspiratory Reserve

7. To measure expiratory reserve, breathe normally several times. After a normal breath has been exhaled, gently blow any remaining air through the mouthpiece. Perform this measurement three times, and compute the average of the resulting volumes.

   Trial 1 _____liters

   Trial 2 _____liters   Average = _____liters

   Trial 3 _____liters   Expiratory Reserve

8. To measure vital capacity, inhale as much air as possible, and gently blow through the mouthpiece. Gently exhale as much air as possible through the mouthpiece. Perform this measurement three times, and compute the average of the resulting volumes.

   Trial 1 _____ liters

   Trial 2 _____ liters   Average = _____ liters

   Trial 3 _____ liters   Vital Capacity

9. Use a colored pen or pencil to chart your results in Figure 20-2. Compare your results with the normal lung volume reading.
10. Why is the average of three volume measurements used to determine the laboratory results?

   _____

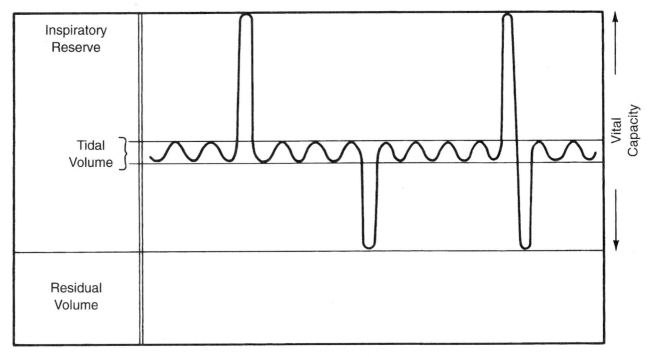

Figure 20-2 Lung volumes.

11. What is the value of your residual volume? Why can't this value be measured?

_____

_____

_____

_____

12. Vital capacity, by definition, is the sum of the inspiratory reserve, tidal volume, and expiratory reserve. Add these three values as they were measured in the laboratory activity. How does this number compare with the volume of the vital capacity that was measured in the activity? Why may these values differ?

Inspiratory Reserve + Tidal Volume + Expiratory Reserve = _____

Measured Vital Capacity = _____

_____

_____

_____

13. Would the vital capacity of an athlete be larger or smaller than that of someone who does not exercise regularly? Explain your answer.

_____

_____

_____

_____

14. List three possible sources of error in this activity.

_____

_____

_____

_____

Teaching Pursed Lip Breathing

Respiratory health professionals are responsible for teaching patients ways to improve their breathing. Practice this exercise, Skill List 20-1, from the textbook, and answer the questions that follow.

Directions

1. Maintain medical asepsis by using the guidelines provided in the Standard and Transmission-Based Precautions, including good handwashing technique and use of gloves as needed.
2. Instruct the patient to assume an upright position such as sitting or standing.
3. Ask the patient to relax the shoulders and neck muscles.
4. Mouth closed, tell the patient to slowly inhale through the nose for at least 2 seconds.
5. Instruct the patient to exhale slowly through tightly pursed lips, as if he or she were gently flickering a candle, but do not force the air out. The exhale should take twice as long as the inhalation (i.e., at least 4 seconds.)
6. Continue to breathe in this manner until breathing returns to normal.

1. Which did you find easier, giving instructions or following instructions?

_____

_____

2. What changes did you notice in yourself when you followed the instructions to perform pursed lip breathing?

_____

_____

_____

_____

3. Did your partner(s) experience similar sensations?

_____

_____

4. What is pursed lip breathing used for?

_____

_____

CRITICAL THINKING

Smoking Choices

The rights of the nonsmoker and smoker have become a source of conflict for many people. Laws have been enacted to protect the nonsmoker from "secondhand" smoke by limiting smoking to designated areas.
Health insurance companies offer lower rates to corporations that offer smoking cessation programs for their employees.

1. Should the rights of nonsmokers be considered more important than those of smokers? Why or why not?

_____

_____

_____

_____

_____

_____

2. Do you believe that a law should be enacted to restrict or eliminate smoking entirely? Explain your answer.

_____

_____

_____

_____

_____

_____

3. Most insurance agencies give a discount for homeowner policies if the occupants are nonsmokers. They do this because statistics indicate that smokers present a higher risk of fires and other household claims. What other factors could be considered by insurance companies to determine rates?

_____

_____

4. Health insurance companies charge higher premiums for smokers than non-smokers. Do you support this policy? Why or why not?

_____

_____

_____

_____

21 Surgical Technologists

CAREERS

Careers, Duties, and Credentials

Using the chapter and other sources, fill in the missing information.

CAREER TITLE	EDUCATION	DESCRIPTION OF JOB DUTIES	LICENSURE	CREDENTIALS
Surgical technologist				
		Manages the heart–lung machine during surgery		

Education Costs and Earnings Potential

Using the Internet, research the educational cost of a surgery-related career and the salary that might be earned in the local area. Use the information to complete the table.

CAREER	INSTITUTION FOR EDUCATION	COST OF EDUCATION	POTENTIAL EARNINGS

Skills and Qualities

Choose a career discussed in the chapter. List three personal qualities and skills that you think are important for the job and the reason(s) why.

1. _____

2. _____

3. _____

KNOWLEDGE CHECK

Multiple Choice

Circle the one correct answer to each of the following questions.

1. Which term means a state of calm?
   a. Anesthesia
   b. Coma
   c. Sedation
   d. Unconscious

2. Donna is a registered nurse who works in the operating room (OR). The time she spends in the OR – before, during and after surgery – is referred to as the
   a. postoperative period.
   b. preoperative period.
   c. perioperative period.
   d. anteoperative period.

3. Which professional is mainly responsible for creating a sterile environment by performing asepsis?
   a. Perfusionist
   b. Surgeon
   c. Perioperative nurse
   d. Scrub tech

4. A _____ regulates blood circulation and composition by administering blood products and anesthetic agents under the direction of the surgeon or anesthesiologist.
   a. scrub tech
   b. perioperative nurse
   c. circulator
   d. perfusionist

5. What is the meaning of the term extracorporeal circuit?
   a. The patient's blood is oxygenated outside the body using a machine.
   b. The patient's respiratory function is handled by a machine.
   c. The patient's blood wastes are extracted and filtered by a machine.
   d. The patient's brain function is measured using a computer.

6. Surgical technologists (STs) can have many roles in the operating room. What was the average annual wage for a ST in the United States in 2019?
   a. $25,300
   b. $31,800
   c. $48,300
   d. $73,800

7. Surgical technologists (STs) can work in hospitals and also outpatient ambulatory care centers. About what percentage of STs work in an outpatient setting?
   a. 20%
   b. 5%
   c. 50%
   d. 85%

8. Rigorous and careful cleaning helps to achieve surgical asepsis. What is another term for surgical asepsis?
   a. Decontamination technique
   b. Cleanliness protocol
   c. Sterile technique
   d. Sterile protocol

9. Which is a medical term meaning free of infectious pathogens?
   a. Clean
   b. Decontaminated
   c. Sanitized
   d. Aseptic

10. During surgical procedures, cutting is a primary action. What is the term for the cutting out or removal of tissue?
    a. Incision
    b. Resection
    c. Ablation
    d. Excision

11. Intentionally destroying tissue in surgery is called
    a. resection.
    b. excision.
    c. ablation.
    d. incision.
12. _____ are used to close a surgical wound.
    a. Retractors
    b. Sutures
    c. Trocars
    d. Hemostatic forceps
13. An endoscope can be flexible or rigid and allows the surgeon to
    a. measure the surgical incision.
    b. keep an open incision clean and dry.
    c. view inside the body.
    d. seal off blood vessels.
14. Which type of surgery is performed with the goal of improving a patient's functional ability, such as a knee replacement?
    a. Cosmetic
    b. Palliative
    c. Restorative
    d. Diagnostic
15. Kayleigh is scheduled for a breast biopsy. Which category of surgery is a biopsy?
    a. Curative
    b. Restorative
    c. Diagnostic
    d. Cosmetic
16. A medical device that sterilizes surgical instruments and supplies is called a(n)
    a. trocar.
    b. autoclave.
    c. centrifuge.
    d. antiseptic.

True/False

Read the following statements and write "T" for true or "F" for false in the blanks provided. If a statement is false, correct the statement to make it true.

_____ 1. At a minimum, a bachelor's degree is required to become a surgical technologist (ST).
_____ 2. Ambulatory surgery centers are also called same-day surgery centers.
_____ 3. The "timeout" before surgery allows the surgical team to make sure everyone knows what is happening, and is required by OSHA.
_____ 4. The medical suffix -scopy means looking into.
_____ 5. Electrosurgery uses electrical current to cauterize, or freeze, tissue.
_____ 6. A surgical procedure to remove an intestinal obstruction would be considered elective surgery in most cases.
_____ 7. A transplant of a smaller organ, such as the pancreas, would be considered major surgery.
_____ 8. Sutures come in a variety of diameters, described with a number of zeroes. The more zeroes, the larger the size.
_____ 9. An autoclave uses ethylene oxide to destroy proteins in microorganisms on medical equipment.
_____ 10. The process of the surgical scrub takes place immediately after gowning and gloving.

Matching

Match the numbered suffix below with its meaning.

1. _____	-ectomy	A. Creation of an opening
2. _____	-rrhaphy	B. Looking into
3. _____	-centesis	C. Repair or suture of
4. _____	-stomy	D. Destruction of
5. _____	-plasty	E. Excision or removal of
6. _____	-opsy	F. Fusion of two parts
7. _____	-lysis	G. Surgical puncture
8. _____	-desis	H. Viewing
9. _____	-scopy	I. Cutting into or incision of
10. _____	-tomy	J. Repair or reconstruction of

Fill in the Blank

Fill in each of the spaces provided with the missing word or words that complete the sentence.

1. A procedure performed primarily to enhance personal appear is considered to be in the _____ category of surgery.
2. A procedure performed to relieve symptoms of a disease process, but not cure it, is in the _____ category of surgery.
3. In surgery, _____ are instruments used to hold tissues aside.
4. Sutures are generally classified according to their materials into two categories: _____ and _____ .
5. _____ surgery is performed in a body cavity or body area through one or more endoscopes, small incisions, cameras, and fiberoptic lighting.
6. Surgical procedures are categorized by the reason for the procedure, the area of the body, the extent of what needs to be done, and the _____ of the procedure.
7. _____ provides the surgeon with visual and manipulation capabilities far beyond the naked eye and human hands.
8. A(n) _____ is a surgical instrument that can puncture and withdraw fluid.
9. _____ uses extreme cold to destroy tissue by freezing it.
10. Precise incisions and simultaneous sealing of blood vessels and nerve endings are advantages of _____ surgery.

PERFORMANCE INSTRUCTION

Effectiveness of Handwashing

Read all directions before beginning this activity. Laboratory activities should be performed under the supervision of a qualified professional only.

Equipment and Supplies

Paper towels
Sink
Scrub brush (optional)
Soap
Antiseptic hand rub
Ultraviolet light indicator
Ultraviolet light

Directions

1. Cover your hands with a spray or lotion that is visible under ultraviolet light only. Allow the solution to dry.
2. Following the skill list procedure found in the textbook, wash and dry your hands with water.
3. Observe your hands briefly under the ultraviolet light to determine whether any indicator was missed. Record your results.
4. Perform the activity again, using soap and water, to compare the effectiveness of this technique in removing the indicator.
5. Observe your hands briefly under the ultraviolet light to determine whether any indicator was missed. Record your results.
6. Perform the activity again, using water, soap, and a surgical scrub brush, to compare the effectiveness of this technique in removing the indicator.
7. Observe your hands briefly under the ultraviolet light to determine whether any indicator was missed. Record your results.
8. Perform the activity again, using antiseptic hand rub, to compare the effectiveness of this technique in removing the indicator.
9. Observe your hands briefly under the ultraviolet light to determine whether any indicator was missed. Record your results.
10. Continue washing your hands, if necessary, until all of the indicator has been removed.
11. Replace all equipment and supplies in the designated area.

Materials Used	Observations
Water only	
Soap and water	
Soap, water, and brush	
Antiseptic hand rub	

Questions

1. Did you wash all areas of your hands equally well? If not, what areas did you miss?

_____

_____

_____

2. Which was the most effective method of hand washing for you?

_____

_____

_____

3. Compare your results with those of your classmates. Did you all observe the same findings?

_____

_____

_____

_____

4. If not, what do you think might account for the differences in your findings?

_____

_____

_____

Sterilizing Packages

Read all the directions before beginning this activity. Sterilization is the process used to kill all microorganisms on an object. Laboratory activities should be completed under the supervision of a qualified professional only.

Equipment and Supplies
Autoclave
Autoclave tape
Autoclave paper or lint-free towel
Metal instrument for sterilization

Directions
1. Maintain medical asepsis by using good handwashing technique. Wrapping packages for sterilization is a clean procedure that requires the hands and instruments to be as free of microorganisms as possible.
2. Select clean instruments for sterilization. Instruments may be arranged into sets for convenient use in particular procedures.
3. Select a wrapping towel or drape that is large enough to cover all contents completely. Drapes for autoclave sterilization may be made of cotton or specialized disposable material. Draping materials must allow penetration by the pressurized steam or gas.
4. Place instrumentation and sterilizing indicator diagonally in the center of the wrapping material. The outside indicating tape does not ensure that the inner contents have been sterilized.
5. Fold the corners of the draping material into the center of the tray. The near edge is folded first, sides next, and the far side last. The package should be neat and tight with no exposed edges of the wrapping material. Tuck the last edge into the pocket formed by the first three sides.
6. Seal the package with indicator tape. Secure the tape so that the package will not be pulled open when the tape is removed.
7. Label the tape with the date and time of sterilization, contents, and the initials of the preparer. Items are not considered sterile indefinitely and must be resterilized if not used within a reasonable length of time.
8. Place the package in the appropriate location for articles needing sterilization or load it into the autoclave.
9. Load clean glassware, instruments, or packages into the autoclave with containers and clasps open. Insert the indicator tape or pellet. Supplies may be wrapped in muslin, paper, nylon, or cellophane or in a sealing package before sterilization. During autoclaving, closed containers may explode as a result of the expansion of trapped air. Clasps must be opened to allow sterilization of all surface areas. Wrappers must be made of material that allows penetration by the steam heat.
10. Close and latch the autoclave door.

11. Steam the items for 20 minutes at 20 pounds of pressure at 275°F. The necessary time for sterilization may differ, depending on the size of the load in the autoclave.
12. Allow the pressure of the autoclave to return to zero before opening the door. The pressure reading must be at zero before opening the autoclave to avoid rapid release of steam and possible injury.
13. Remove the sterile equipment or packages and store them in the appropriate location. Individually sterilized articles must be removed with another sterile instrument to prevent contamination.

Questions

1. Why is it important to place a sterilization indicator inside the package as well as outside?

_____

_____

_____

2. Ethylene oxide gas is used to sterilize materials such as plastics and rubber. Why is steam sterilization not used for these materials?

_____

_____

CRITICAL THINKING

Surgical Conscience

Maintaining surgical asepsis in the operating room is an important task. It demands focus, attention to detail, and specialized knowledge. It also requires "surgical conscience." Surgical conscience is the commitment of all personnel in the surgical area to immediately report any violation of the sterile field so that it can be addressed or corrected. This must happen whether anyone else has observed the violation.

1. Why is maintaining asepsis in the operating room so important?

_____

_____

_____

2. What might happen if the sterile field is violated?

_____

_____

_____

3. Imagine you are a surgical technician working with a notoriously bad-tempered surgeon. You notice your coworker has inadvertently breached the sterile field in what you consider a very minor way. Would you report the violation? If not, why not?

_____

_____

_____

4. If you would report the violation in the scenario above, what would you do and say?

_____

_____

_____

5. Do you think it would be difficult to immediately report an error you made yourself? Why or why not?

_____

_____

_____

6. Can you think of any circumstances in which it might be acceptable to not report a violation of the sterile field during surgery?

_____

_____

_____

22 Physical and Occupational Therapy Careers

CAREERS

Careers, Duties, and Credentials

Using the chapter and other sources, fill in the missing information.

CAREER TITLE	EDUCATION	DESCRIPTION OF JOB DUTIES	LICENSURE	CREDENTIALS
		Designs, selects materials, produces, instructs on use, and evaluates appliances that replace limbs		
		Performs nonmedical tasks, prepares hot and cold packs, and helps patients with movement exercises	Not licensed	
	Master's degree and at least 24 weeks of supervised clinical work	Uses activities to help a person develop, maintain, or regain skills that enable satisfying and independent living		
Kinesiotherapist			Not licensed	

Education Costs and Earnings Potential

Using the Internet, research the educational cost of a physical or occupational therapy career and the salary that might be earned in the local area. Use the information to complete the table.

CAREER	INSTITUTION FOR EDUCATION	COST OF EDUCATION	POTENTIAL EARNINGS

Skills and Qualities

Choose a career discussed in the chapter. List three personal qualities and skills that you think are important for the job and the reason(s) why.

1. _____

2. _____

3. _____

Multiple Choice

Circle the one correct answer to each of the following questions.

1. An occupational therapist is likely to concerned with how well a patient can perform basic tasks involving self-care, known as
   a. activities of daily living (ADLs).
   b. core chores of life (CCLs).
   c. fundamental daily tasks (FDTs).
   d. essential life duties (ELDs).

2. Which healthcare professional is in primary care?
   a. Speech language pathologist
   b. Family physician
   c. Cardiovascular surgeon
   d. Physical therapist

3. An occupational therapist usually practices _____ care, typically needing a physician referral to be seen.
   a. primary
   b. secondary
   c. tertiary
   d. quaternary

4. Which level of education is needed by physical therapy assistants?
   a. High-school diploma
   b. Associate degree
   c. Bachelor's degree
   d. Doctoral degree

5. In a larger practice, which of these tasks would be most likely performed by a physical therapy technician?
   a. Developing a plan for the patient
   b. Giving a therapeutic massage
   c. Consulting with patient's PCP
   d. Ordering supplies

6. A kinesiotherapist is a health professional specializing in
   a. assessing a patient's ability to perform ADLs.
   b. designing and fabricating braces and splints.
   c. body movement through exercise.
   d. providing care to patients using artificial limb(s).

7. A patient would see a pedorthist if she were seeking care for her
   a. misaligned spine.
   b. prosthetic leg.
   c. malformed feet.
   d. painful knee.

8. Which body structure(s) are measured when conducting an electromyogram?
   a. Brain
   b. Heart
   c. Muscles
   d. Nerves

9. When a physical therapist is observing a patient's gait, the patient must be
   a. walking.
   b. talking.
   c. thinking.
   d. rotating.

10. The range of motion (ROM) of a patient is measured by the physical therapist with a
    a. speedometer.
    b. scale.
    c. caliper.
    d. goniometer.

11. What is the directional term for when a limb moves closer to another limb?
    a. Flexion
    b. Rotation
    c. Abduction
    d. Pronation
12. What is the term for the downward or backward movement of a hand or foot?
    a. Abduction
    b. Flexion
    c. Pronation
    d. Supination
13. _____ is an intervention performed by a physical therapist.
    a. Surgery
    b. Family counseling
    c. Transcutaneous electrical nerve stimulation
    d. Sonography
14. Which of these is an example of an instrumental activity of daily living (IADL)?
    a. Toileting
    b. Showering
    c. Eating
    d. Managing finances
15. Which assessment tool for physical and occupational therapists is web-based and measures the quality of treatments instead of the total amount of treatment?
    a. Lower Extremity Function Scale (LEFS)
    b. Canadian Occupational Performance Measure (COPM)
    c. Focus on Therapeutic Outcomes (FOTO)
    d. Patient-Specific Functional Scale (PSFS)

True/False

Read the following statements and write "T" for true or "F" for false in the blanks provided. If a statement is false, correct the statement to make it true.

____ 1. Kinesiotherapists work under the supervision and direction of a physician.

____ 2. Certified orthotists design, fabricate, and fit braces, splints, and strengthening apparatuses, which are called orthoses.

____ 3. Physical therapy assistants are not permitted to provide manual therapy, such as therapeutic massage, to patients.

____ 4. Some schools offer accelerated physical therapy programs that allow a student to complete the entire educational requirements in 2 to 3 years.

____ 5. Even entry-level practice as a physical therapist requires a doctoral degree in physical therapy.

____ 6. A prosthetist designs and fits artificial limbs.

____ 7. The word occupation in occupational therapy can refer to any activity the patient considers to be central in their identity.

____ 8. Short wave diathermy is the application of cold to decrease pain, edema, and metabolism.

____ 9. Passive range of motion (PROM) refers to how much a patient's joint can be moved by another external force.

____ 10. The Canadian Occupational Performance Measure is an objective test based on the average of patients with similar conditions.

CONTENT INSTRUCTION

Understanding the Concepts

Using your own words, answer each question in three or four sentences.

1. As understood in the context of occupational therapy, what are two of your most important occupations? Why?

_____

_____

_____

Chapter **22** **Physical and Occupational Therapy Careers**

_____

_____

_____

_____

2. What are some of your daily activities that demonstrate active range of motion?

_____

_____

_____

_____

_____

_____

_____

Illustrating the Concepts

Using stick figures or more elaborate drawings, as you are able, illustrate each of the following pairs of body movements.
1. Flexion and extension
2. Abduction and adduction
3. Pronation and supination

PERFORMANCE APPLICATIONS

Using a Goniometer

Read all of the instructions before beginning this activity. Laboratory activities should be completed under the supervision of a qualified professional only.

Equipment and Supplies

Goniometer

Directions

1. Wash hands thoroughly.
2. Familiarize yourself with the goniometer.
3. Put the center (or fulcrum) of the goniometer at the center of the elbow.
4. Hold the goniometer's stationary arm along the forearm.
5. Have the "patient" stretch the elbow to the points of full flexion and extension.
6. Use the goniometer's moving arm to align with the forearm at both flexion and extension, keeping its center at the center of the elbow.

Measurements

1. Record the range of motion, in degrees, of extension and flexion.
   a. Extension:

   _____

   b. Flexion:

   _____

2. What range of findings did your class observe?

a. Extension:

_____

b. Flexion:

_____

CRITICAL THINKING

Living with Disabilities

According to the Centers for Disease Control and Prevention, 26% of adults in the United States have some type of disability. Disabilities include those of mobility (13.7%), cognition (10.8%), independent living (6.8%), hearing (5.9%), vision (4.6%), and self-care (3.7%). Adult Americans living with disability are much more likely than adults without disabilities to smoke and/or have heart disease, diabetes, and/or obesity.

1. Why do you think the prevalence of smoking and the diseases mentioned above are so much higher among people living with disabilities?

_____

_____

_____

_____

_____

_____

_____

2. What are some variables that influence whether a person living with a disability is able to function at their highest potential?

_____

_____

_____

_____

_____

_____

_____

3. What do you feel is an appropriate way to speak with adult patients living with disabilities about their disabilities? Or do you think that is inappropriate under any circumstances? Why?

_____

_____

_____

_____

_____

_____

_____

4. Do you think a person with limited mobility or self-care ability would appreciate or resent help with tasks, such as putting on a coat, crossing the room, or lifting books? Why?

_____

_____

_____

_____

_____

_____

_____

23 Diagnostic Imaging Careers

Careers, Duties, and Credentials

Using the chapter and other sources, fill in the missing information.

CAREER TITLE	EDUCATION	DESCRIPTION OF JOB DUTIES	LICENSURE	CREDENTIALS
				American Registry of Radiologic Technologists (ARRT)
	Bachelor's degree plus completion of an accredited program			Certification after passing the MDCB exam
Sonographer			Required in 4 states	
Cardiovascular technologist	Associate degree			
		Uses medical imaging and radiation to diagnose and treat disease and injury	Licensed in 50 states	
		Uses sophisticated equipment to record the activity of the brain and nervous system to help diagnose neurological disorders		Certification exam through one of several professional exams

Education Costs and Earnings Potential

Using the Internet, research the educational cost of one diagnostic imaging career and the salary that might be earned in the local area. Use the information to complete the table.

CAREER	INSTITUTION FOR EDUCATION	COST OF EDUCATION	POTENTIAL EARNINGS

Skills and Qualities

Choose a career discussed in the chapter. List three personal qualities and skills that you think are important for the job and the reason(s) why.

1. _____

2. _____

3. _____

177

Multiple Choice

Circle the one correct answer to each of the following questions.

1. What is contrast media?
   a. A type of film used for radiographs
   b. The disc or device where image data is stored
   c. An agent used to make internal structures of the body more visible on radiographs
   d. The opposite of an image; left versus right

2. The subspecialty of radiology that uses imaging to guide surgical procedures is
   a. radiation oncology.
   b. interventional radiology.
   c. procedural radiology.
   d. diagnostic radiology.

3. Which healthcare professional is responsible for administering liquid contrast media?
   a. Radiographer
   b. Laboratory technician
   c. Registered nurse
   d. Radiologist

4. Sam plans on becoming a radiologist and just graduated high school. If he is 18 years old, how old will Sam likely be when he is board eligible – or able to sit for the board exam?
   a. 21–22 years old, depending on specialty
   b. 26–29 years old, depending on specialty
   c. 29–33 years old, depending on specialty
   d. 26–30 years old, depending on specialty

5. Which attribute would most benefit a radiographer?
   a. Writing skills
   b. Mathematical aptitude
   c. Public speaking abilities
   d. Leadership qualities

6. Which healthcare profession requires the most education and experience?
   a. Radiographer
   b. Sonographer
   c. Radiologist
   d. Interventional radiologist

7. Which imaging modality uses sound waves to produce diagnostic images of internal structures of the body?
   a. Computed tomography
   b. Radiography
   c. Sonography
   d. DEXA scanning

8. Nuclear medicine involves the patient swallowing or injecting a _____ that gives off particles which are detected and turned into an image.
   a. contrast medium
   b. positron
   c. radiolucent fluid
   d. tracer

9. What type of energy is used when producing mammograms?
   a. Gamma rays
   b. Radio waves
   c. Sound waves
   d. Ionizing radiation

10. What is the name for the test that records the electrical activity of the heart using electrode pads place on the patient's body?
    a. Electroencephalogram
    b. Echocardiograph
    c. Electrocardiograph
    d. Vascular sonograph

11. What is another name for a sonographer?
    a. X-ray technician
    b. Ultrasound technician
    c. Radiographic technologist
    d. Neurodiagnostic technician

12. What type of imaging produces real-time, moving images?
    a. Arteriography
    b. Computed Tomography (CT)
    c. Nuclear Medicine (NM)
    d. Fluoroscopy

13. In sonography, which term describes the brightest areas?
    a. Isoechoic
    b. Hypoechoic
    c. Hyperechoic
    d. Anenchoic

14. Magnetic resonance imaging (MRI) and computed tomography (CT) both produce detailed images, but MRIs are better for showing
    a. detail of musculoskeletal areas.
    b. clarity of bones and fractures.
    c. contrast of soft tissue.
    d. blood flow issues.

15. What is revealed by a DEXA scan?
    a. Fractures
    b. Blood flow
    c. Bone density
    d. Lung capacity

16. A chest X-ray exposes a patient to about 0.0001 grays (Gy) of radiation. What is the typical dosage of radiation that is used when attacking a solid tumor?
    a. 0.040–0.080 grays
    b. 10.0–20.0 grays
    c. 4.0–10.0 grays
    d. 40–80 grays

17. Which body plane is the midline?
    a. Frontal
    b. Sagittal
    c. Oblique
    d. Medial

18. Which body plane cuts the superior and inferior sections?
    a. Oblique
    b. Transverse
    c. Sagittal
    d. Frontal

19. Which directional terms means something is nearer?
    a. Distal
    b. Lateral
    c. Superior
    d. Proximal

20. _____ is a directional term that refers to something above.
   a. Superior
   b. Lateral
   c. Proximal
   d. Distal

True/False

Read the following statements and write "T" for true or "F" for false in the blanks provided. If a statement is false, correct the statement to make it true.

_____ 1. In diagnostic imaging, the term modality refers to the settings on the X-ray machine.

_____ 2. Imaging professionals, such as radiographers, position patients, obtain images, and construct initial diagnoses.

_____ 3. DEXA is usually performed on the lower spine and hips.

_____ 4. Near-infrared spectroscopy (NIR) is a technique that allows noninvasive measuring of cerebral functions.

_____ 5. Positron emission tomography (PET) sends high-frequency soundwaves from a handheld transducer into the patient's body.

_____ 6. X-rays are blocked by radiopaque structures such as bones and teeth while softer tissues are said to be radiolucent.

_____ 7. The term supine means a patient is on their back facing up.

_____ 8. According to radiation safety precautions, exposure should be as long as restrictions allow (ALARA).

_____ 9. Persons under the age of 18 are not permitted to work with radiation.

_____ 10. The Occupational and Safety Administration (OSHA) limits employees' radiation exposure to a certain level annually.

CONTENT INSTRUCTION

Abbreviations

Match each of the following abbreviations with the phrase that best describes its meaning or function. Then write the phrase or name for each of the abbreviations in the spaces provided.

Abbreviation	Meaning or Function
1. _____ CT	a. Test to monitor the electrical activity of the heart
2. _____ EEG	b. Technique that revolutionized imaging by using computers with radiographs
3. _____ EKG	c. Detailed image produced using a magnetic field
4. _____ MRI	d. Noninvasive technique using light to measure cerebral function
5. _____ NIR	e. Uses computers and radiography to visualize metabolic activities
6. _____ PET	f. Measures electrical activity of the brain

1. CT:_____

2. EEG:_____

3. EKG:_____

4. MRI:_____

5. NIR:_____

6. PET:_____

Research

1. Explore and describe three common contrast media used in imaging.

_____

_____

_____

_____

_____

_____

Image I-dentification

Identify the imaging modality used to produce each image.

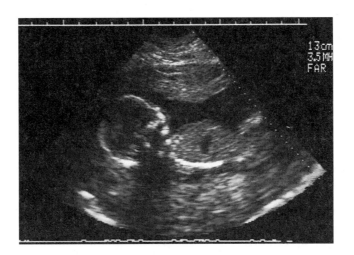

1. _____

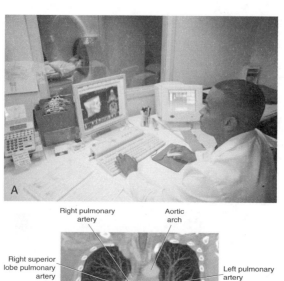

Right pulmonary artery — Aortic arch

Right superior lobe pulmonary artery — Left pulmonary artery

Right middle lobe pulmonary artery — Left superior lobe pulmonary artery

— Left superior pulmonary vein

Right inferior lobe pulmonary artery

B

Right inferior pulmonary vein — Left atrium

(**A**, From Fuse/Thinkstock; **B**, from Long B, Rollins J, Smith B: *Merrill's atlas of radiographic positioning and procedures*, ed 13, St. Louis, 2016, Mosby.)

2. _____

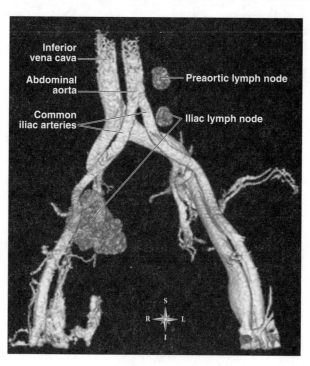

Inferior vena cava — Preaortic lymph node

Abdominal aorta

Common iliac arteries — Iliac lymph node

S
R — L
I

(From Patton KT, Thibodeau GA: *Anatomy & physiology*, ed 9, St. Louis, 2016, Mosby.)

3. _____

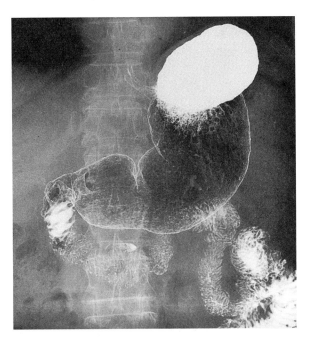

(From Lampignano JP, Kendrick LE: *Bontrager's textbook of radiographic positioning and related anatomy*, 9th ed., St. Louis, 2018, Elsevier.)

4. _____

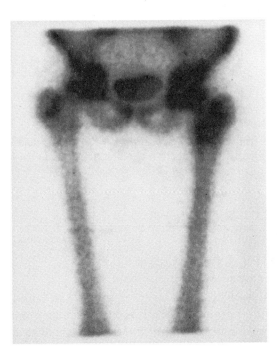

(From Baker A, Macnicol MF: Haematogenous osteomyelitis in children: epidemiology, classification, aetiology and treatment, *Paediatr Child Health* 18(2):75-84, 2008.)

5. _____

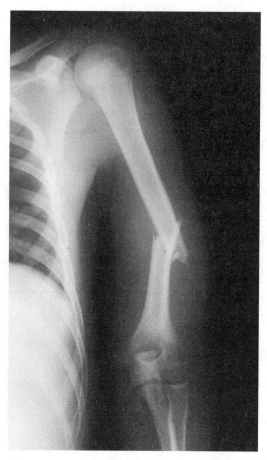

(From Long B, Rollins J, Smith B: *Merrill's atlas of radiographic positioning and procedures*, ed 13, St. Louis, 2016, Mosby.)

6. _____

PERFORMANCE APPLICATIONS

Determining the Effect of Light Rays

Light and radiographic waves come from the same electromagnetic spectrum and share many of the same properties. Work in groups of two or three for this activity. Read all of the directions before beginning the activity. Laboratory activities should be completed under the supervision of a qualified professional only.

Equipment and Supplies

Construction paper (optional), flashlight, penlight, yardstick

Directions

1. Hold a flashlight perpendicular to the wall at a distance of 1 foot.
2. Measure the diameter of the image produced by the beam on the wall.
3. Repeat the procedure, holding the flashlight 2, 3, 4, and 5 feet from the wall. Record the results.
4. Repeat steps 1 through 3, using the penlight as the energy source. Record the results.
5. Using the flashlight as the energy source, repeat steps 1 through 3 while holding a piece of construction paper 6 inches from the wall between the wall and beam of the flashlight during all measurements. Record the results.

Questions

1. How does the area covered by the beam from the light source that is near the wall compare with the area covered at a greater distance?

_____

_____

_____

_____

_____

2. Was the beam produced by the light source stronger or weaker in intensity as it was moved farther from the wall?

_____

_____

_____

_____

_____

3. Why does the operator of radiographic equipment maintain as great a distance from the beam as possible?

_____

_____

_____

_____

_____

4. How does the construction paper placed between the light source and the wall represent the action of a lead shield used in radiography?

_____

_____

_____

_____

_____

CRITICAL THINKING

Using your own words, answer each question in two or three sentences.

1. Your friend says that he would never work in radiology because he does not want to become sterile from exposure to radiation. What should you say?

_____

_____

_____

_____

_____

_____

185

2. Your friend tells you she is not going to have mammograms taken because she believes she will get cancer from the radiographs. What should you say?

_____

_____

_____

_____

_____

_____

3. List the advantages and disadvantages of one medical imaging occupation including the following factors: job opportunities, salary range, fringe benefits, working conditions, occupational hazards, and educational requirements.

_____

_____

_____

_____

_____

_____

_____

_____

_____

_____

_____

_____

24 Phlebotomists and Dialysis Technicians

Careers, Duties, and Credentials

Using the chapter and other sources, fill in the missing information.

CAREER TITLE	EDUCATION	DESCRIPTION OF JOB DUTIES	LICENSURE	CREDENTIALS
Phlebotomist			None	
		Set up and run dialysis machines; perform venipuncture; monitor patients during dialysis	None	
Blood bank specialist				

Education Costs and Earnings Potential

Using the Internet, research the educational cost of one of the careers in this chapter and the salary that might be earned in the local area. Use the information to complete the table.

CAREER	INSTITUTION FOR EDUCATION	COST OF EDUCATION	POTENTIAL EARNINGS

Skills and Qualities

Choose a career discussed in the chapter. List three personal qualities and skills that you think are important for the job and the reason(s) why.

1. _____

2. _____

3. _____

KNOWLEDGE CHECK

Multiple Choice

Circle the one correct answer to each of the following questions.

1. The area of the arm, anterior to the elbow, where blood is typically drawn from is called the _____ space.
   a. antecubital
   b. medial
   c. flexor
   d. cannula

2. Which of these body systems is a network of arteries and veins that moves blood throughout the body?
   a. Renal system
   b. Integumentary system
   c. Vascular system
   d. Endocrine system

3. Sara is enrolled in an accelerated phlebotomy program, hoping to complete her training in the least amount of time. How long will her training last?
   a. 2 years
   b. 1 year
   c. 3 months
   d. 7.5 weeks

4. Which healthcare professional's duties include selecting donors, blood typing, and pretransfusion testing?
   a. Phlebotomist
   b. Blood bank specialist
   c. Dialysis technician
   d. Pathologists' assistant

5. Patients with dysfunctional kidneys who cannot properly filter waste out of their blood are treated with a process called
   a. transfusion.
   b. centrifuge.
   c. dialysis.
   d. fractionation.

6. Which healthcare professional may complete a 12- to 18-month certification from the Nephrology Nursing Certification Commission (NNCC)?
   a. Blood bank specialist
   b. Phlebotomist
   c. Dialysis technician
   d. Apheresis phlebotomist

7. Why do medical professionals almost always draw blood from veins rather than arteries?
   a. Veins carry richer blood and produce better quality samples than arteries.
   b. Veins are easily accessed and not under pressure like arteries.
   c. Veins make easier targets because they are typically thicker and further away from the surface of the skin.
   d. Veins are under pressure, resulting in a quicker process.

8. In order to test blood samples as whole blood, a technician will operate a(n) _____ to separate the sample into solid and liquid portions.
   a. evacuated tube
   b. centrifuge
   c. splitter
   d. plasma table

9. After a blood sample is separated by the centrifugation process, which formed elements are at the bottom?
   a. White blood cells
   b. Red blood cells
   c. Plasma
   d. Platelets

10. The buffy coat within a blood sample is a mixture of
    a. white blood cells and platelets.
    b. red blood cells and platelets.
    c. red and white blood cells.
    d. plasma and platelets.

11. Ethylenediaminetetraacetic acid (EDTA) is the anticoagulant found in the _____-topped tube.
    a. red
    b. tiger
    c. green
    d. lavender

12. Anticoagulants may be added to an evacuated tube to prevent clotting and platelet clumping. What is the term for the liquid that has not been treated with this anticoagulant?
    a. Serum
    b. Plasma
    c. Whole blood
    d. Buffy coat

13. Federal law mandates that all newborns be screened for _____ and phenylketonuria between 24 and 72 hours after birth.
    a. diabetes
    b. hypothyroidism
    c. sickle cell anemia
    d. vitamin K deficiency

14. What is the goal of the fractionation process?
    a. To isolate proteins from plasma
    b. To separate whole blood into solids and liquid
    c. To filter out malignant white blood cells
    d. To draw blood at high volume

15. Of the four major blood types, which is considered the universal recipient due to its lack of reactive antibodies?
    a. B
    b. AB
    c. A
    d. O

16. The process that filters waste from body fluid using a membrane in the abdomen is called
    a. gastric dialysis.
    b. hemodialysis.
    c. peritoneal dialysis.
    d. gravitational dialysis.

17. What is the first step in the chain of custody quality control process?
    a. Centrifuge
    b. Sample collection
    c. Requisition
    d. Chromatography

18. The _____ requires employers to provide personal protective equipment (PPE), such as gloves, gowns, and masks, to phlebotomists.
    a. Occupational Health and Safety Administration (OSHA)
    b. National Nephrology Certification Commission (NNCC)
    c. National Phlebotomy Association (NPA)
    d. Commission of Office Laboratory Accreditation (COLA)

True/False

Read the following statements and write "T" for true or "F" for false in the blanks provided. If a statement is false, correct the statement to make it true.

_____ 1. Phlebotomy and venipuncture refer to the same thing.

_____ 2. Blood bank specialists and phlebotomists both draw blood; however, blood bank specialists must have at least a baccalaureate degree accredited by the Commission on Accreditation of Allied Health Education Programs (CAAHEP) and certification as a medical technologist.

_____ 3. Evacuated tubes can have additives, which are represented by the color of the stopper.

_____ 4. The butterfly method is preferred by phlebotomists when drawing blood from larger veins and arteries.

_____ 5. Venipuncture is the procedure used when only small amounts of blood are required for testing.

_____ 6. Mr Tynes was told by his physician that he possesses the rare Rh antigen. This antigen is found in the red blood cells of less than half of North Americans.

_____ 7. Some lifestyle changes that can be experienced by a patient receiving dialysis are weight gain and trouble sleeping.

_____ 8. The quality control process during venipuncture begins with the sealing and labeling of the patient's blood sample.

_____ 9. The Bloodborne Pathogen Standard requires used needles to be discarded in a red biohazardous waste bag.

_____ 10. After obtaining the required blood samples, the phlebotomist uses an elastic band called a tourniquet to stop the venipuncture site from bleeding.

Understanding Blood Types

1. Using the chapter and other sources, fill in the missing information.

BLOOD TYPE	CAN DONATE BLOOD TO:	CAN RECEIVE BLOOD FROM:
A		
B		
AB		
O		

2. Review the Blood Typing section in the textbook, then access this website and follow the directions there to play a blood typing simulation game.
   http://www.nobelprize.org/educational/medicine/bloodtypinggame/game/index.html

Evaluating Dialysis

Research the different types of dialysis. One good source is the National Kidney Foundation, referenced under Advocacy and Research in the textbook. Answer the following questions.

1. Where did you research the information about different types of dialysis?

_____

_____

_____

2. List the pros and cons of each type of dialysis.
   a. Hemodialysis

_____

_____

_____

_____

_____

_____

_____

   b. Peritoneal dialysis

_____

_____

_____

_____

_____

_____

_____

Chain of Custody

The chain of custody documents where a specimen has been and the persons who handled it. Inaccurate results from misplacing or misidentifying a patient sample can be a legal matter in the case of drug testing and DNA analysis and may harm or cause death in the patient if a diagnosis is missed or blood chemistry improperly analyzed.

Equipment and Supplies

Paper and pencil or pen, computer with Internet access, printer

Directions

1. Without using the Internet, consider the points at which a blood specimen may require documentation in the chain of custody. Make a list of possibilities, and include the title of the person who would be involved at each step.
2. Develop your own chain of custody form, including the information you compiled in step 1 of this exercise.
3. Using the Internet, find sample chain of custody forms. Print one.

Drawing Conclusions

1. What points and people were on your initial list for the chain of custody?

_____

_____

_____

_____

_____

2. How was the form you developed similar to the chain of custody form you printed? How did it differ?

_____

_____

_____

_____

_____

_____

_____

3. What parts of the form you printed surprised you?

_____

_____

_____

_____

_____

_____

_____

4. Where did you find the form you printed?

_____

5. Describe a scenario in which the chain of custody is broken. What consequences might there be in that case?

_____

_____

_____

_____

_____

_____

_____

_____

_____

Venipuncture Supplies

Identify each lettered object in the image.

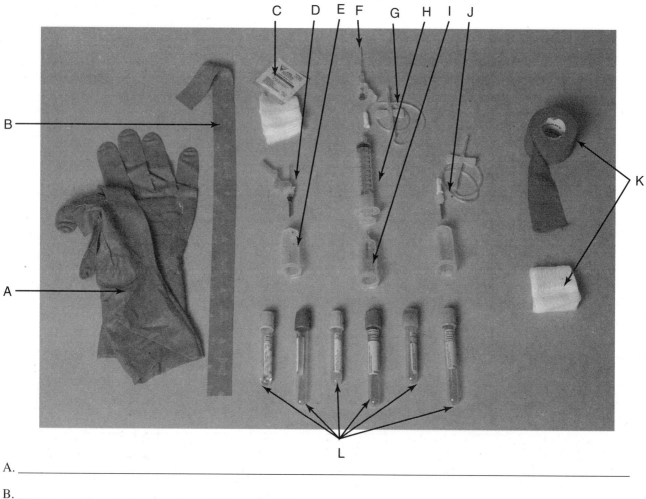

A. _____

B. _____

C. _____

D. _____

E. _____

F. _____

G. _____

H. _____

I. _____

J. _____

K. _____

L. _____

CRITICAL THINKING

Needle Phobia

Needle phobia, or the extreme fear of needles and medical procedures involving needles, is surprisingly common. It is estimated that 10% of Americans experience this fear. Because people with this phobia may be reluctant to seek medical attention if they think it will involve the use of needles, the phobia can negatively impact sufferers' health.

1. Do you know anyone who has a needle phobia? If so, what has been their experience when confronted with the prospect of having their blood drawn?

   _____

   _____

   _____

2. How do you think a needle phobia develops?

   _____

   _____

   _____

   _____

   _____

   _____

3. Imagine you are a phlebotomist. What could you do to help an anxious patient?

   _____

   _____

   _____

   _____

   _____

   _____

   _____

193

Dialysis

As you learned in your research about hemodialysis and peritoneal dialysis, there are advantages and disadvantages to each. If you were in the position of needing dialysis and you were able to choose one or the other, which type of dialysis would you choose? Why?

_____

_____

_____

_____

_____

_____

Plasmapheresis

Donor plasmapheresis is the process in which a quantity of the donor's blood is removed, the plasma is separated from red blood cells, and the blood cells are returned to the donor. Plasma from donors is used in medical therapies to treat patients with rare disorders, such as primary immunodeficiency disease, Kawasaki disease, and hemophilia A. It is also used to treat patients who have experienced burns, trauma, shock, animal bites, and liver conditions, among other conditions.

It usually takes between 1 and 3 hours to donate plasma, and people can donate twice within a 7-day period (although there are restrictions on the number of times a donor can undergo plasmapheresis annually).

1. Why do you think some people might choose to donate plasma?

_____

_____

_____

_____

_____

_____

2. What are some reasons a person would choose not to donate plasma?

_____

_____

_____

_____

_____

3. Some private companies offer compensation to donors who undergo plasmapheresis. Why do you think that is the case?

_____

_____

_____

_____

_____

_____

4. Do you think providing compensation for plasma is a good idea? Why or why not?

_____

_____

_____

_____

_____

_____

_____

25 Clinical Laboratory Careers

CAREERS

Careers, Duties, and Credentials

Using the chapter and other sources, fill in the missing information.

CAREER TITLE	EDUCATION	DESCRIPTION OF JOB DUTIES	LICENSURE	CREDENTIALS
				MLT
		Studies the chemical nature of living things. Analyzes and researches the effects of hormones, enzymes, serums, and foods on the tissues and organs of animals		
	Minimum of an associate degree is required. Candidates can also choose more advanced training in the field where they study biology or a related science in a 4-year program, then enroll in a master's program for 2 more years of coursework and clinical rotations.			PA(ASCP)
Microbiologist			Licensure not required	
Pathologist				Various certifications available
				MT(ASCP)
Medical laboratory assistant				Various certifications available

Education Costs and Earnings Potential

Using the Internet, research the educational cost of one clinical laboratory career and the salary that might be earned in the local area. Use the information to complete the table.

CAREER	INSTITUTION FOR EDUCATION	COST OF EDUCATION	POTENTIAL EARNINGS

197

Skills and Qualities

Choose a career discussed in the chapter. List three personal qualities and skills that you think are important for the job and the reason(s) why.

1. _____

2. _____

3. _____

KNOWLEDGE CHECK

Multiple Choice

Circle the one correct answer to each of the following questions.

1. A microorganism that can cause disease is known as
   a. pathogenic.
   b. nonpathogenic.
   c. contagious.
   d. benign.

2. In response to a newspaper article exposing the failure by labs to detect cervical cancer, which regulations were developed by Congress in 1988?
   a. Laboratory Quality Act (LQA)
   b. Clinical Laboratory Improvement Amendments (CLIA)
   c. Health Insurance Portability and Accountability Act (HIPAA)
   d. Corrective Measures of Labs Act (CMLA)

3. What is a pathologist?
   a. A medical doctor specializing in human reproduction
   b. A medical professional who studies the spread of disease in a population
   c. A medical professional who collects samples from a patient
   d. A medical doctor who examines specimens to diagnose disease

4. Which professional specializes in the preparation and study of tissue samples?
   a. Immunotherapist
   b. Hematologist
   c. Histotechnologist
   d. Cytotechnologist

5. Maria is examining cells from a patient's liver under a microscope. What type of medical laboratory scientist is she?
   a. Cytotechnologist
   b. Immunologist
   c. Chemist
   d. Hematologist

6. Which professional is responsible for calibrating laboratory equipment and running quality control tests?
   a. Medical laboratory scientist
   b. Cytologist
   c. Histologist
   d. Pathologist

7. Which type of microbiologist uses the body's own defense mechanisms to fight disease?
   a. Virologist
   b. Immunologist
   c. Geneticist
   d. Pathologist

8. What is a test that studies the physical and chemical characteristics of the urine?
   a. Blood film
   b. Urinalysis
   c. Reagent
   d. Toxicology

9. What is agar?
   a. A machine that spins samples at high speeds
   b. A way to test equipment accuracy
   c. A substance used to culture or reproduce microorganisms
   d. The subject of analysis in the lab

10. Mr Martin's doctor is concerned he may have diabetes and has ordered lab tests to monitor his glucose. In the lab, Mr Martin's blood sample is exposed to a substance that produces a chemical reaction. What is the term for this other substance?
    a. Analyte
    b. Reagent
    c. Substrate
    d. Blood film

11. Upon receiving the results of his blood test, Mr Dobbs noticed his hemoglobin level was 15.5 grams per deciliter (g/dL). His doctor told him the value was normal because it fell between two predetermined values. What is the term for these two values?
    a. Reference range
    b. Value chart
    c. Value span
    d. Normalcy span

12. What is the study of poisons?
    a. Microbiology
    b. Biochemistry
    c. Toxicology
    d. Pathology

13. The _____ time is how long it takes a solute to pass through a chromatography column during a toxicology test.
    a. retention
    b. completion
    c. conversion
    d. elongation

14. What laboratory technique sorts molecules by size?
    a. Electrophoresis
    b. Centrifugation
    c. Automation
    d. Chain of custody

15. How long can blood be stored if frozen?
    a. Up to 1 month
    b. Up to 3 months
    c. Up to 1 year
    d. Up to 3 years

16. Quality assurance processes in laboratories aim to make sure
    a. the same test would yield the same results regardless of who performs it.
    b. better trained individuals get better results.
    c. testing is performed as soon as possible.
    d. the results can be read by laypersons, especially patients.

17. What is the term for the quality control process that ensures are specimen will be tested properly and without contamination?
    a. Chain of custody
    b. Chain of causation
    c. Specimen control map
    d. Sample control chain

18. A given test is known to have a 95% sensitivity, meaning that
    a. 95% of the tests will return a false negative.
    b. 5% of the tests will return a false negative.
    c. 95% of the tests will return a false positive.
    d. 5% of the tests will return a false positive.

True/False

Read the following statements and write "T" for true or "F" for false in the blanks provided. If a statement is false, correct the statement to make it true.

_____ 1. An analyte is a substance used in testing that produces a chemical reaction in the presence of the substance being tested.

_____ 2. Medical laboratory technologists (MLTs) require an associate degree and one year in a medical laboratory science (MLS) program.

_____ 3. Some accomplishments of microbiological research include the development of vaccines for polio and other diseases.

_____ 4. Laboratory personnel perform liquid chromatography (LC) to measure the number and types of blood cells in the patient's sample.

_____ 5. Pathogenic microorganisms growing and multiplying in the body result in a state of disease called infection.

_____ 6. The Centers for Disease Control and Prevention (CDC) waives CLIA compliance for certain tests where an erroneous result is highly unlikely and which pose little risk to the patient.

_____ 7. Electrophoresis is used to identify disease processes that might create abnormal proteins, to detect antibodies that indicate the body is responding to infection, and to study DNA.

_____ 8. Another name for a blood film test is a blood smear.

_____ 9. An analyte is made of nutrients such as seaweed, potatoes, or blood and is used in the laboratory as something microorganisms can grow on.

_____ 10. Specificity measures a test's ability to accurately give negative results for people who do not have the condition under testing.

CONTENT INSTRUCTION

Understanding the Concepts

Answer the questions about the laboratory tests discussed in the textbook.

1. What is the name of the test that measures the following analytes: sodium, potassium, chloride, calcium, creatinine, blood urea nitrogen, glucose, and glycosylated hemoglobin?

   _____

   _____

   _____

2. What is the difference between gas chromatography and liquid chromatography? What does chromatography do?

   _____

   _____

   _____

   _____

3. Name four of the nine organisms discussed in the textbook that can cause disease in humans.

   _____

   _____

   _____

   _____

4. Of the organisms listed in the previous answer, which group is the most common cause of human disease and infection?

   _____

   _____

5. A hematologist puts a blood sample in a centrifuge. In your own words, explain what happens to the sample.

_____

_____

_____

6. What hematological test preparation might be used to assist in the diagnosis of leukemia?

_____

_____

7. What analyte is used in a specific gravity test? What does a specific gravity test measure?

_____

_____

_____

PERFORMANCE APPLICATIONS

Using the Microscope to Identify Microorganisms

Review the directions for use of the microscope found in the textbook in Skill List 25-4. You will be assigned a microorganism or secretion specimen by your teacher. Read all of the directions before beginning this activity. Laboratory activities should be completed under the supervision of a qualified professional only.

Equipment and Supplies

Cover slip
Eyedropper
Microscope
Microscope slide
Prepared slide of microorganism
Unknown specimen
Water

Directions

1. Maintain medical asepsis by practicing good handwashing technique.
2. Follow the directions for microscope use to observe and draw the prepared slide under low, medium, and high power.
3. Prepare a wet mount slide (Skill List 25-5 in the text) by placing a small amount of the unknown specimen in the center of a clean slide. Add a drop of water to the specimen if it is not already in a solution.
4. Cover the specimen with a clean cover slip.
5. Follow the directions for microscope use to observe and draw the prepared slide under low, medium, and high power.
6. Clean and return all materials to the designated location.

Drawing Conclusions

1. How does the field of vision, or amount of the specimen, compare when the microscope is switched from low to high power?

_____

_____

_____

_____

_____

2. Why is it important to look at the objective from the side when moving it toward the stage?

_____

_____

_____

_____

_____

3. What does parfocal mean?

_____

_____

_____

_____

_____

Identifying Microorganisms in the School and Home Environment

Review the information in the textbook regarding preparation of sterile agar plates and transfer of bacteria (Skills Lists 25-1 and 25-2) before beginning this activity. Many bacteria can be found in common household and school environments. Read all of the directions before beginning this activity. Laboratory activities should be completed under the supervision of a qualified professional only.

Equipment and Supplies

Autoclave or bleach
Grease pencil or China marker
Incubator
Sterile culture swab
Sterile nutrient agar plate

Directions

1. Maintain medical asepsis by practicing good handwashing technique.
2. Prepare a sterile agar plate and culture swab. A wooden cotton swab can be sterilized for use as a culture swab.
3. Collect a specimen by rubbing the cotton swab on a surface in your environment. Do not allow the cotton swab to touch any other surface.
4. Open the sterile plate to inoculate the agar with the culture swab. Close the plate immediately.
5. Discard the culture swab in the proper receptacle.
6. Mark the bottom of a sterile agar plate with the site of specimen collection, date, and your initials.
7. Place the closed plate in an incubator at 37°C. Place the plate upside down to prevent condensation or liquid from forming on the specimen.
8. Incubate the plate for 3 or 4 days. Make observations for each 24-hour period.
9. Count the number of different types of bacterial colonies on the plate. Create a data chart or drawing to record your results.
10. Compare your results with other locations in the environment.
11. To prevent the spread of unknown microorganisms, sterilize or disinfect the agar before discarding it.
12. You may repeat the procedure by testing for airborne microorganisms only. For this activity, the plate should be exposed to the air in different locations for a designated length of time before incubation.
13. Clean and return all materials to the designated location.

Drawing Conclusions

1. How many and what type of bacterial colonies did your plate show after incubation?

_____

_____

_____

_____

2. In what area of the environment did your class find the most bacterial growth?

_____

_____

_____

_____

3. Why do you think it is important to sterilize or disinfect the culture plates before discarding them?

_____

_____

_____

_____

4. Why do you think is 35–36°C used for incubation of the microorganisms?

_____

_____

_____

_____

5. Why do you think the bacteria could not be seen before incubation?

_____

_____

_____

_____

Urinalysis

Read all of the directions before beginning this activity. Urine composition may be determined through a series of simple tests. Disposable gloves are worn for handling body secretions. Laboratory activities should be completed under the supervision of a qualified professional only.

Equipment and Supplies

Chemical "dipstick" indicator strip with reference chart
Hydrometer or graduated cylinder with urinometer
Natural or artificial urine
Paper or urine specimen cup
pH paper (or similar acid/base indicator) with reference chart

Directions

1. Collect the appropriate type of urine specimen needed for each test.
2. Observe the clarity of a fresh, routine specimen of urine. Record the appearance.

_____

3. Note the odor of a fresh, routine specimen of urine. Describe this smell.

_____

4. Perform a pH test using a fresh, routine specimen of urine. Litmus, Nitrazine, or hydrion paper may be used as an indicator. Each paper turns varied colors in acidic and basic solutions. Dip the bottom half of a small piece of indicator paper in the specimen. Compare the color of the paper with the chart provided with the paper. Do not touch the paper container with the urine-soaked paper while comparing the colors. Record the value of the pH of the urine.

_____

5. Perform a specific gravity test using a fresh, routine specimen of urine. Pour the urine into a graduated cylinder or hydrometer container to a level 1 inch below the top of the cylinder. Without touching the sides of the cylinder, gently twist and release the urinometer into the urine. Read the results of the specific gravity as soon as the spinning stops. Record the value of the specific gravity.

_____

6. Use "dipsticks" to determine the presence of any abnormal components of urine, including blood, sugar, acetone, and proteins. Follow the manufacturer's instructions for the use of each indicating stick. Record the presence of any abnormal components.

_____

Drawing Conclusions

Characteristic	Normal	Abnormal
Volume	1–1.5 L/day	Polyuria (>2.0 L/day) Oliguria (<0.5 L/day)
Odor	None	Sweet (sugar) Ammonia (old) Offensive (bacteria)
Color	Yellow, straw, amber	Red (blood, infection, some drugs) Brown (bile) Orange, blue (drugs)
Turbidity	Clear	Cloudy (pus, bacteria, cells, fat, phosphates)
pH	4.8–7.4 (average 6)	Alkaline (phosphates, vegetarian diet)
Specific gravity	1.002–1.04	High (dehydration) Low (diuresis)

Abnormal Component	Possible Cause
Sugar (glycosuria)	Diabetes mellitus
Protein (albuminuria)	Renal disease
Ketones (ketonuria)	Incomplete fat metabolism, diabetes mellitus
Blood (hematuria)	Infection, injury
Pus (pyuria)	Infection
Bacteria (bacteriuria)	Infection
Casts	Dead cells, injury

1. Use the table to determine whether the observation of clarity made in Step 2 is normal. If the value is outside of the normal range, why might it be different?

_____

_____

2. Use the table to determine whether the odor noted in Step 3 is normal. If the value is outside of the normal range, why might it be different?

_____

_____

3. In Step 4, the directions state that care should be taken not to touch the pH paper container with the urine-soaked paper. Why is this important?

_____

_____

4. Use the table to determine whether the value obtained for the pH is normal. If the value is not within the normal range, why might it be different?

_____

_____

5. Use the table to determine whether the value obtained for the specific gravity is normal. If the value is not within the normal range, why might it be different?

_____

_____

_____

6. Use the table to determine what the presence of any abnormal components in the urine specimen might mean, and describe the condition.

_____

_____

_____

_____

CRITICAL THINKING

1. You are going to draw blood for laboratory tests. You ask your patient if he has been fasting. He says that he has had nothing except coffee with cream and no sugar. What should you say?

_____

_____

_____

_____

2. Your friend tells you that she had laboratory work done a week earlier, and because no one has called, she assumes everything is fine. What should you say?

_____

_____

_____

3. You are going to draw blood for laboratory tests. Your patient tells you that she is extremely afraid of needles. What should you do?

_____

_____

_____

_____

26 Biotechnology Research and Development Professionals

CAREERS

Careers, Duties, and Credentials

Using the chapter and other sources, fill in the missing information.

CAREER TITLE	EDUCATION	DESCRIPTION OF JOB DUTIES	LICENSURE	CREDENTIALS
Genetic counselor				Via the American Board of Genetic Counseling (ABGC)
Biological/ laboratory/research technician or technologist				
Geneticist				
		Design, develops, and helps maintain instruments and machines that are used to monitor and treat disease in health care		Available

Education Costs and Earnings Potential

Using the Internet, research the educational cost of one of the biotechnology research and development careers discussed in this chapter, and the salary that might be earned in the local area. Use the information to complete the table.

CAREER	INSTITUTION FOR EDUCATION	COST OF EDUCATION	POTENTIAL EARNINGS

Skills and Qualities

Choose a career discussed in the chapter. List three personal qualities and skills that you think are important for the job and the reason(s) why.

1. _____

2. _____

3. _____

Multiple Choice

Circle the one correct answer to each of the following questions.

1. Biotechnology applies scientific techniques to the manipulation of the _____ of living organisms for human purposes.
   a. brain
   b. nerves
   c. blood
   d. genes

2. Which government entity develops laboratory safety guidelines?
   a. Food & Drug Administration (FDA)
   b. Centers for Disease Control and Prevention (CDC)
   c. Department of Agriculture (USDA)
   d. National Center for Biotechnology Information (NCBI)

3. Dr Rita Colwell classified each branch of biotechnology by color in 2003. Which color corresponds to medicine and health?
   a. Blue
   b. Green
   c. Red
   d. Yellow

4. *Most* biomedical engineers and bioengineers work in which setting?
   a. Government
   b. Manufacturing
   c. Hospitals
   d. Clinics

5. The interdisciplinary field of _____ combines biology, computer science, and information technology for study.
   a. bioinformatics
   b. genetics
   c. microbiology
   d. immunology

6. Which type of medical biotechnologist studies patterns of inheritance to treat disorders?
   a. Immunologist
   b. Microbiologist
   c. Biophysicist
   d. Geneticist

7. Biological technicians work under the supervision of the scientist and help with many procedures, as well as cleaning and sterilizing equipment. What is the educational requirement for an entry-level biological technician?
   a. High-school diploma
   b. Bachelor's degree
   c. Master's degree
   d. Master's degree plus internship

8. Which type of research performed by biomedical scientists purposely sets out to solve a particular problem?
   a. Pure research
   b. Fundamental research
   c. Basic research
   d. Applied research

9. What is the term for variation within a gene?
   a. Gamete
   b. Mutation
   c. Allele
   d. Autosome

10. Human chromosomes are paired and referred to as homologous
    a. phenotypes.
    b. genotypes.
    c. autosomes.
    d. gametes.

11. Genes are segments of _____ found within nucleus of the cell.
    a. chromosomes
    b. messenger RNA (mRNA)
    c. deoxyribonucleic acid (DNA)
    d. transfer RNA (tRNA)
12. How many pairs of chromosomes exist in the nucleus of every cell in humans?
    a. 12 pairs
    b. 23 pairs
    c. 46 pairs
    d. 72 pairs
13. The nucleic acid of the deoxyribonucleic acid (DNA) are _____ -based and attach to sugar and phosphate.
    a. hydrogen
    b. oxygen
    c. glucose
    d. nitrogen
14. What is the study of how to arrange reproduction within a human population to increase the occurrence of heritable characteristics regarded as desirable?
    a. Gene mapping
    b. Epigenetics
    c. Congenics
    d. Eugenics
15. The cells harvested from a zygote are _____, which are able to differentiate into more specialized cells.
    a. stem cells
    b. nerve cells
    c. transfer RNA
    d. messenger RNA
16. The most common technique to edit genes is called
    a. genome modifying protocol (GMP).
    b. clustered regularly interspaced short palindromic repeats (CRISPR).
    c. nonhomologous end-joining (NHEJ).
    d. long palindromic ribonucleic modification (LPRM).
17. What is the name for proteins that can be engineered to bind to target molecules on cells for therapeutic purposes during immunotherapy?
    a. Monoclonal antibodies
    b. Messenger RNA
    c. Transfer RNA
    d. Vectors
18. DNA is extracted from the nucleus of a cell through a process called
    a. genome extraction.
    b. helix reduction and isolation.
    c. cell lysis.
    d. nucleic refraction.
19. What does the electrophoresis process do?
    a. Splits and isolates DNA's helixes
    b. Sends genetic information to cells
    c. Sorts base pairs of DNA so they are visible to the naked eye
    d. Replaces abnormal genes with new or edited versions
20. In cytogenetics, what is the term for the visual representation of an individual's chromosomes?
    a. Genetic map
    b. Karyotype
    c. Agarose
    d. Karyogram

True/False

Read the following statements and write "T" for true or "F" for false in the blanks provided. If a statement is false, correct the statement to make it true.

_____ 1. In 1972, Stanford researchers were the first to cut DNA from different species and join them together, inventing the process called CRISPR.

_____ 2. The study of how genes are expressed in ways other than the structural DNA sequence is called epigenetics.

_____ 3. The body process of meiosis creates two identical cells by cell division.

_____ 4. A polyclonal antibody (pAB) is a laboratory-produced antibody derived from cloned cells.

_____ 5. A genetic trait that will not appear unless it is carried by both parents' chromosomes is referred to as recessive.

_____ 6. Suppression immunotherapy works by engaging the immune system to act on a disease.

_____ 7. Most genetic disorders are multifactorial.

_____ 8. Electrophoresis allows the laboratory personnel to detect and measure antibodies, antigens, and other proteins in a sample.

_____ 9. Enzyme-linked immunosorbent assay technique (ELISA) is a method of DNA preparation used in a wide range of testing, genomic, and engineering applications.

CONTENT INSTRUCTION

Identifying the Structure of DNA

Label the diagram of DNA in Figure 26-1.

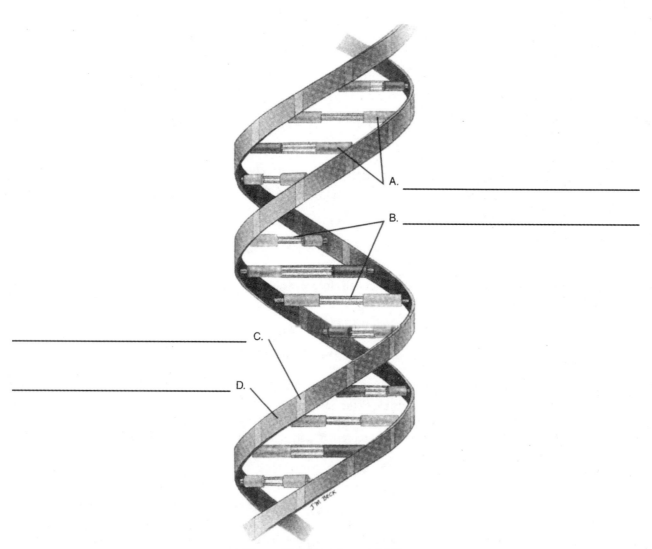

Figure 26-1 Structure of DNA.

A. _____

B. _____

C. _____

D. _____

Determining Probability of Inheritance

Cystic fibrosis is often used to study hereditary traits because a recessive, autosomal gene carries it. Cystic fibrosis results in the inadequate production of certain enzymes. The condition is characterized by too much mucus in the lungs. It can be detected by testing for salt on the skin. Treatment includes eating a diet that is high in protein and calories. The person with this condition also must use good pulmonary hygiene, which may include postural drainage, to keep the lungs free of excess secretions. Postural drainage involves positioning the body to drain secretions into the bronchi so that they may be removed or excreted by coughing. Antibiotics are used to treat infections if they occur. People with cystic fibrosis may live well past middle age with proper care.

Cystic fibrosis is the most commonly occurring recessive disorder in the white population.

The probability of inheriting a genetic disorder may be determined using a Punnett square. In the example of cystic fibrosis, the parents may have a genetic configuration of genotype as follows:

Father's Genotype   Mother's Genotype

    Ff   Ff

Both parents are carriers. That means that they both carry the recessive gene (f) for cystic fibrosis, but they do not have the condition themselves because the gene is recessive. Having the dominant gene (F) means that the phenotype, or appearance, of each of these individuals is not to have cystic fibrosis.

During meiosis, or sexual cell reproduction, the sperm and egg of the mother and father are formed using one of the genes possible for this trait. The chances of the sperm and egg containing the F or the f gene are exactly equal.

The Punnett square can be used to determine the probability that the offspring will show the condition of cystic fibrosis. The square is formed by placing the father's genes on top and the mother's genes on the side, as shown in the Punnett square below.

The probability of the offspring having the condition of cystic fibrosis (genotype ff) is one in four, or 1/4. The probability of the offspring being a carrier (genotype Ff) is two in four, or 1/2.

1. Complete the Punnett square shown below to determine the probability of a couple showing the following genotypes producing an offspring with cystic fibrosis. The father's phenotype is that he has the condition (genotype ff). The mother is a carrier (genotype Ff).

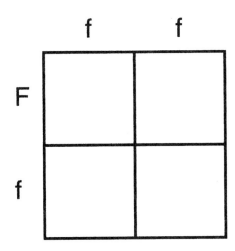

a. The probability of the offspring having cystic fibrosis (genotype ff) is _____ in four, or _____%.
b. The probability of the offspring being a carrier (genotype Ff) is _____ in four, or _____%.
c. The probability of the couple producing a child without the condition is _____ in four, or _____%.

2. Complete the Punnett square shown below for a couple who has the following phenotypes. The father is a carrier (genotype Ff). The mother does not carry this recessive gene (genotype FF).

a. The probability of the offspring having cystic fibrosis (genotype ff) is _____ in four, or _____%.
b. The probability of the offspring being a carrier (genotype Ff) is _____ in four, or _____%.
c. The probability of the couple producing a child without the condition is _____ in four, or _____%.

3. Why is the probability of the second child showing the condition of cystic fibrosis for the couple in Question 1 the same as the probability of their first child having this genetic configuration?

_____

_____

_____

4. Why is the probability of the sperm containing the F or f gene exactly the same when the father's genotype is Ff?

_____

_____

_____

PERFORMANCE APPLICATIONS

Performing a DNA Extraction

Read all of the directions before beginning this activity. Laboratory activities should be completed under the supervision of a qualified professional only.

Equipment and Supplies

Alcohol
250-mL beaker
Dishwashing liquid
Eyedropper
Glass rod
Hot water bath
Nonpathogenic bacteria (yeast may be used)
Nutrient broth (water for yeast)
    Test tube
    Test tube holder
    Thermometer

Directions

1. Maintain medical asepsis by practicing good handwashing technique.
2. Prepare a broth of nonpathogenic bacteria or mix yeast in water at 50°–60°C.
3. Pour approximately 10 mL of bacterial broth into a clean test tube.
4. Add approximately 5 mL of dishwashing liquid to the test tube.
5. Place the test tube in a hot water bath for 15 minutes. Do not exceed 60°C.
6. Use an eyedropper to add alcohol to cover the top of the solution.
7. Gently stir a glass rod into the solution through the alcohol.
8. Continue to stir the glass rod through the alcohol into the solution.
9. Record your observations.
10. Clean materials as directed by your instructor, and place them in the designated location.

Drawing Conclusions

1. What are the fibers called that collect around the glass tube?

_____

2. Why must the glass rod be turned gently in the solution?

_____

_____

_____

3. What is the purpose of each of the reagents used in the extraction?

_____

_____

_____

_____

_____

Karyotype Online Simulation

Use the following Internet link to simulate genetic disorders due to karyotype abnormalities. Complete the karyotype for each of the three patients.
University of Arizona Biology Project:
http://www.biology.arizona.edu/human_bio/activities/karyotyping/karyotyping.html

Questions

1. What notation would you use to characterize Patient A's karyotype?

_____

2. What diagnosis would you give Patient A?

_____

3. What notation would you use to characterize Patient B's karyotype?

_____

4. What diagnosis would you give Patient B?

_____

5. What notation would you use to characterize Patient C's karyotype?

_____

6. What diagnosis would you give Patient C?

_____

CRITICAL THINKING

Harvest of Fear

Use the PBS NOVA website called "Harvest of Fear" to investigate genetically modified foods. Prepare a position report either for or against the use of genetically modified foods. Print and complete the video worksheet from the teachers' activity page while researching the website or watching the video (if available). Choose one of the character roles to play and complete the "Are Genetically Modified Foods Safe?" from the teachers' activity page. Hold a debate from the point of view of your role using the information gathered. If the video is not available, use the Internet to research the answers to the questions.

PBS: http://www.pbs.org/wgbh/harvest/

Summarize your opinion about the use of genetically modified foods.

_____

_____

_____

_____

_____

_____

_____

_____

_____

_____

_____

_____

Stem Cells

Research using stem cells focuses on understanding how diseases occur and how those diseases can be treated with the use of stem cells. Some of the diseases that might benefit from stem cell therapies include Parkinson's disease, heart disease, spinal cord injuries, cancer, ALS, and Alzheimer's disease. The use of stem cells remains controversial, however, largely because they are often obtained, with permission, from early-stage embryos from in vitro fertilization clinics.

Make two arguments, one in favor of stem cell research and one opposed to it. Then, disclose which is your actual opinion, and why.

Stem cell research should not be allowed because:

_____

_____

_____

_____

Stem cell research should be allowed because:

_____

_____

_____

_____

_____

_____

Regarding stem cell research, I believe it should:

_____

_____

_____

_____

_____

_____

Exercises in Genetic Counseling

Consider the following situations that might occur in a genetic counseling center. Describe what action you feel would be appropriate for the counselor to follow.

1. The patient comes in for testing to determine whether her fetus inherited two genes for cystic fibrosis. Testing is done on the woman and her husband. The blood tests show that the fetus does have the condition but that the husband is not a carrier. The woman forbids the counselor from telling the husband that the child is not his. How would you respond if you were the genetic counselor?

_____

_____

2. Two patients have the genetic condition polydactyly. They want their fetus tested for the condition. They inform the counselor of their intention to abort any fetus that is "normal," or without the condition. They feel that they do not want to raise a child who is different from them. How would you respond if you were the genetic counselor?

_____

_____

3. A patient carries the genetic trait for sickle cell anemia. She tells you that she will abort any fetus that carries the gene, because she wants the condition to end with her generation. How would you respond if you were the genetic counselor?

_____

_____

_____

27 Speech Language Pathologists and Audiologists

CAREERS

Careers, Duties, and Credentials

Using the chapter and other sources, fill in the missing information.

CAREER TITLE	EDUCATION	DESCRIPTION OF JOB DUTIES	LICENSURE	CREDENTIALS
	At least two years of study and 100 hours of supervised clinical experience		Must practice under a licensed SLP	
		Performs tasks as delegated by an audiologist, including those that facilitate patient flow in the office		C-AA
Otolaryngologist			Licensed by state	
Speech language pathologist				
Audiologist				CCC-A, ABA® Certified, PASC®, CISC®

Education Costs and Earnings Potential

Using the Internet, research the educational cost of a speech language pathology or audiology career and the salary that might be earned in the local area. Use the information to complete the table.

CAREER	INSTITUTION FOR EDUCATION	COST OF EDUCATION	POTENTIAL EARNINGS

Skills and Qualities

Choose a career discussed in the chapter. List three personal qualities and skills that you think are important for the job and the reason(s) why.

1. _____

2. _____

3. _____

KNOWLEDGE CHECK

Multiple Choice

Circle the one correct answer to each of the following questions.

1. Which term means *pertaining to the sense of hearing*?
   a. Auditory
   b. Dysphagia
   c. Audiogram
   d. Apraxia

2. Audiologists can help determine reasons for _____, or dizziness.
   a. dysphagia
   b. vertigo
   c. dysarthria
   d. aphasia

3. What is the main role of a speech-language pathologist?
   a. To diagnose and treat hearing and balance problems
   b. To diagnose and treat language problems
   c. To treat ailments of the oral cavity
   d. Teaching English to non-English speakers

4. Which part(s) of the body do otolaryngologists diagnose and treat?
   a. The lungs and the larynx
   b. The back, hips, and legs
   c. The ears, nose, and throat
   d. The oral cavity

5. What is the main role of an audiologist?
   a. To diagnose and treat disorders and diseases of the ear, nose, and throat
   b. To diagnose and treat hearing and balance disorders
   c. To diagnose and treat language problems
   d. To assist speech-language pathologists

6. Which professional would be most likely to send out hearing aids for repair, receive fixed devices, coordinate with insurers and payers, and generally facilitate patient flow in the office?
   a. Audiologist
   b. Speech-language pathologist assistant
   c. Otolaryngologist
   d. Audiology assistant

7. What level of education is required for audiologists to practice in their state?
   a. Bachelor's degree
   b. Bachelor's degree plus certification
   c. Associate degree plus 500 hours of shadowing a certified audiologist
   d. Doctoral degree

8. What is the purpose of an Individualized Family Service Plan, which is prepared by a speech-language pathologist for a child under 3 years old?
   a. Documenting strengths and services and improving communication and function of the child
   b. Ensuring proper insurance reimbursement
   c. Keeping the child's health record accurate and up to date
   d. To submit to the parent's for billing purposes

9. What is the meaning of the term aphasia?
   a. The inability to speak
   b. Difficulty swallowing
   c. Dysarthria
   d. Echolalia

10. Mrs Bachman suffered a stroke last year and sees a speech-language pathologist to treat her _____, or difficulty swallowing.
    a. dysphagia
    b. aphasia
    c. apraxia of speech
    d. dysarthria

218

11. What is the name for a small unit of sound that is made to distinguish one word from another?
    a. Consonant
    b. Vowel
    c. Phoneme
    d. Voice

12. Which is true of the phoneme /v/?
    a. It is voiced.
    b. It is a plosive.
    c. It is bilabial.
    d. It is velar.

13. The inner ear contains a series of canals called bony _____, which includes the cochlea, semicircular canals, and vestibule.
    a. eustachian tubes
    b. endolymph
    c. saccule
    d. labyrinth

14. Most people notice hearing loss when they cannot understand normal speech or they develop _____, which is a ringing in the ear.
    a. apraxia
    b. dysarthria
    c. tinnitus
    d. anacusis

15. What is the name of the middle ear bacterial or viral infection, which is common in young children?
    a. Tinnitus
    b. Otitis media
    c. Vertigo
    d. Otosclerosis

16. Unlike a hearing aid, a cochlear implant does not amplify sound, but instead stimulates the
    a. auditory nerve.
    b. hammer and anvil.
    c. hair cells.
    d. inner ear fluid.

17. Maha's client, 2-year-old Jackson, has been diagnosed with childhood-onset fluency disorder. Jackson's parents have been taking him to see Maha every Friday to improve his dysfluency. What type of health professional is Maha?
    a. A speech-language pathologist (SLP)
    b. An otolaryngologist (ENT)
    c. An audiologist
    d. An audiology assistant

18. Dr Stevens has a patient with a dual-diagnosis mental disorder. One of the characteristics of the patient's disorder is that he automatically repeats what another person has said. What is this condition called?
    a. Auditory apraxia
    b. Dysarthria
    c. Dysphagia
    d. Echolalia

19. What is audiometry?
    a. Measurement of the range and sensitivity of a person's hearing
    b. Measurement of a person's vocal ability
    c. An instrument used to view the structures of the ear
    d. A method of plotting frequency and volume

20. What is an otoscope?
    a. A device that measures accuracy of hearing
    b. A device that measures balance or equilibrium
    c. An instrument used to view the structure of the ear
    d. An instrument used to record speech

True/False

Read the following statements and write "T" for true or "F" for false in the blanks provided. If a statement is false, correct the statement to make it true.

_____ 1. An IFSP is a documented assessment of the school-age child's current function, how it affects the child's education, and the services and accommodations the child will require.

_____ 2. Anacusis is a term meaning *a unit of sound*.

_____ 3. Certification for audiologists is voluntary.

_____ 4. An audiologist is a medical doctor.

_____ 5. The entry level of practice for speech-language pathologists is a master's degree.

_____ 6. Patients with social (pragmatic) communication disorder and patients with autism spectrum disorder (ASD) each have difficulty communicating appropriately in a social manner; the key difference is that patient with ASD tends to be more outgoing.

_____ 7. People with Wernicke's aphasia can say words, but their brain does not connect the sound to concepts.

_____ 8. Aphasia is a motor speech disorder in which weakened muscles or dysfunctional communication between the brain and facial muscles results in poor speech.

_____ 9. Communication skills are divided into receptive abilities, such as hearing words and sounds and understanding what they mean, and expressive abilities—that is, being able to talk.

_____ 10. An audiometer emits specific sounds of varying frequency, which are measured in decibels.

CONTENT INSTRUCTION

Fill in the Chart

Fill in the missing information about normal language milestones.

BEHAVIOR	RECEPTIVE/EXPRESSIVE ABILITY?	AGE WHEN BEHAVIOR APPEARS
Uses 2- to 3-word "sentences" to talk about and ask for things		
Pays attention to music		
Tells stories that stick to a topic		
Cries differently for different needs		
Responds to changes in tone of your voice		
Points to pictures in a book when named		
Uses many different consonant sounds at the beginning of words		
Usually understood by people outside the family		
Enjoys games such as peekaboo and pat-a-cake		

Fill in the Blank

Fill in each of the spaces provided with the missing word or words that complete the sentence.

1. Sensorineural hearing loss (SNHL) results from damage to cochlea or _____ _____.

2. The primary function of the ear is the _____ sense.

3. A(n) _____ is an electronic device used to treat profound deafness and severe hearing loss.

4. The semicircular canals of the inner ear contain a clear fluid called _____.

5. _____ is the insertion of tubes to relieve pressure and fluid from the middle ear.

6. Another name for the tympanic membrane of the ear is the _____.

7. _____ is a bacterial or viral infection of the middle ear that is common in young children.

8. A(n) _____ is a device that treats hearing loss through the amplification of sound.

9. Sound waves may be transmitted through the _____ bone, or fluid.

10. Besides hearing, a second function of the ear is to help maintain _____.

PERFORMANCE APPLICATIONS

Care of Hearing Aids

Hearing aids are devices that act as miniature loudspeakers to make sounds louder. The hearing aid does not cure the hearing impairment. It requires proper care and maintenance to be effective. Hearing aids may be worn:

- In the ear
- Behind the ear
- Behind the ear with a plastic tube leading into the ear canal
- Built into eyeglasses
- Clipped to the wearer's clothing with a cord and button-like receiver in the ear

Simple guidelines to use when speaking to an individual wearing a hearing aid as well as steps for care of the hearing aid are:

- Face the person directly when speaking.
- Speak clearly, slowly, and naturally.
- Do not place the hearing aid in direct sunlight or on hot surfaces.
- Do not use hair spray while the hearing aid is in place.
- Do not get the hearing aid wet.
- Clean the ear mold by carefully removing wax with a pipe cleaner or toothpick.
- Wash the ear mold in mild soap and water if it can be detached from the hearing aid.
- Inspect the tubing for cracks, loose connections, and twisting, which may indicate the need for replacement.

Questions

1. Would it be necessary to speak loudly to a person wearing a hearing aid?

_____

_____

_____

2. Why is it important to remove the hearing aid before taking a shower or bath?

_____

_____

_____

3. Rubbing alcohol has the property of drying materials. Why is it important to avoid the use of it when cleaning hearing aids?

_____

_____

_____

Researching Resources

Choose an advocacy and research organization from those listed in the textbook. Use the Internet to explore the website of your chosen organization. Determine the following information.

1. What organization did you choose?

_____

2. What is the organization's mission?

_____

_____

_____

_____

3. What are two resources the organization offers to individuals and/or families of individuals?

_____

_____

_____

_____

_____

_____

4. What are two resources the organization offers to professionals?

_____

_____

_____

_____

_____

CRITICAL THINKING

Deaf Culture

The conviction that deafness is a form of human experience rather than a disability underlies the structure of Deaf culture. Members of communities that embrace Deaf culture share an identity with history and norms around deafness as it is experienced and expressed through arts, social institutions, values, and language (in this case, sign language).

A 2000 documentary, The Sound and the Fury, portrayed the conflict between two sets of parents in an extended family. Each set of parents had a child born deaf. One family elected to have a cochlear implant installed in their infant; the other family, members of Deaf culture, chose not to have a cochlear implant installed in their child.

222

Use the Internet to research Deaf culture, and answer the following questions.

1. Discuss why someone might choose to embrace deafness as a source of identity and community.

_____

_____

_____

_____

_____

2. Discuss why a parent might reject the installation of a cochlear implant in an infant.

_____

_____

_____

_____

_____

3. Discuss why someone might reject the concept of Deaf culture.

_____

_____

_____

_____

_____

Working with Children with Development Language Disorders

In working with a child with a developmental language disorder, a speech-language pathologist has a number of interventions available. These include natural approaches, such as playing alongside the child and talking about what is happening, and more structured techniques, such as drills.

The textbook includes a number of examples of common interventions. Review those and then answer these questions.

1. Of the interventions described in the textbook, which do you think would be most challenging to use? Why?

_____

_____

_____

_____

_____

_____

_____

2. What factors do you think influence the effectiveness of the interventions?

_____

_____

_____

_____

_____

_____

_____

_____

28 Dieticians and Nutritionists

Careers, Duties, and Credentials

Using the chapter and other sources, fill in the missing information.

CAREER TITLE	EDUCATION	DESCRIPTION OF JOB DUTIES	LICENSURE	CREDENTIALS
	Bachelor's degree plus internship currently; master's degree as on 1/1/2024			
Nutritionist		Varied and undefined		
Certified Nutrition Specialist				
Dietetic technician				

Education Costs and Earnings Potential

Using the Internet, research the educational cost of one of the nutrition-related careers discussed in this chapter, and the salary that might be earned in the local area. Use the information to complete the table.

CAREER	INSTITUTION FOR EDUCATION	COST OF EDUCATION	POTENTIAL EARNINGS

Skills and Qualities

Choose a career discussed in the chapter. List three personal qualities and skills that you think are important for the job and the reason(s) why.

1. _____

2. _____

3. _____

Multiple Choice

Circle the one correct answer to each of the following questions.

1. Beginning in 2024, the Commission on Dietetic Registration (CDR) will require which level of education by a student in order to sit for the RD or RDN exam?
   a. High-school diploma
   b. Associate degree
   c. Bachelor's degree
   d. Master's degree

2. A registered dietician (RD) is qualified to provide _____ and, in 13 states, is the only practitioner of nutrition allowed to do so.
   a. macronutrient therapy (MNT)
   b. medical nutrition therapy (MNT)
   c. micronutrient therapy (MNT)
   d. modern nutrient teaching (MNT)

3. The average national annual wage for a Registered Dietician (RD) in 2019 was between
   a. $130,000 and $135,000.
   b. $10,000 and $25,000.
   c. $25,000 and $35,000.
   d. $60,000 and $65,000.

4. A patient with a colostomy has a(n) _____ through which waste exits the body.
   a. aperture
   b. stoma
   c. G-tube
   d. rectad

5. What are lipids?
   a. Red blood cells
   b. Enzymes
   c. Fats
   d. Hormones

6. What is the name for the body process of breaking down tissue?
   a. Parental nutrition
   b. Catabolism
   c. Anabolism
   d. Enteral nutrition

7. Which is an example of a micronutrient?
   a. Fat
   b. Protein
   c. Fiber
   d. Calcium

8. Which nutrient is the main source of immediate energy for the body?
   a. Protein
   b. Fat
   c. Carbohydrates
   d. Cholesterol

9. Which nutrient slows down digestion by expanding into a gel in water?
   a. Saturated fat
   b. Unsaturated fat
   c. Insoluble fiber
   d. Soluble fiber

10. Which nutrients are organic and regulate cell metabolism?
    a. Minerals
    b. Vitamins
    c. Enzymes
    d. Hormones

11. Which calculation determines body mass index (BMI)?
    a. height × weight = BMI
    b. weight ÷ height = BMI
    c. weight ÷ age = BMI
    d. age ÷ weight = BMI
12. A patient who has lost her sense of taste entirely is experiencing
    a. anosmia.
    b. dysgeusia.
    c. ageusia.
    d. stoma.
13. The provider records that Jim has anosmia, meaning that he cannot
    a. taste food.
    b. digest food.
    c. smell food.
    d. swallow food.
14. Which type of nutrition support is being applied when a patient is receiving nutrients directly into their bloodstream by intravenous (IV) administration?
    a. Partial nutrition (PN)
    b. Parenteral nutrition (PN)
    c. Entire nutrition (EN)
    d. Enteral nutrition (EN)
15. The FDA's reference daily intake (RDI) is used to determine the Daily Value (DV) for consumers. How many calories per day is the DV based on?
    a. 1,000
    b. 1,500
    c. 2,000
    d. 2,500
16. What is the final step in the nutrition care process (NCP)?
    a. Nutrition diagnosis
    b. Nutrition monitoring and evaluation
    c. Nutrition assessment
    d. Nutrition intervention
17. During which of the four steps in the nutrition care process (NCP) would blood tests likely be completed?
    a. Nutrition monitoring and evaluation
    b. Nutrition intervention
    c. Nutrition assessment
    d. Nutrition diagnosis
18. Which of these therapeutic diets might be recommended for a patient with colitis or stomach ulcer?
    a. Low calorie
    b. Low fat
    c. Bland
    d. High protein
19. Which vitamin deficiency can result in slowed blood clotting?
    a. Vitamin C
    b. Vitamin D
    c. Vitamin E
    d. Vitamin K
20. Which diet is most likely to be recommended for diabetics?
    a. High protein
    b. High calorie
    c. Low carbohydrate
    d. Low fat

True/False

Read the following statements and write "T" for true or "F" for false in the blanks provided. If a statement is false, correct the statement to make it true.

_____ 1. You meet a woman on the subway who introduces herself as a nutritionist and hands you a business card. Because "nutritionist" is a protected title requiring licensure, you can be sure she has obtained at least a master's degree.

_____ 2. Most dietitians and nutritionists work in hospitals and other institutional settings, such as nursing homes.

_____ 3. Dietetic technicians may work independently or under the supervision of an RD.

_____ 4. All the essential amino acids can be found in plant food sources as they provide complete proteins.

_____ 5. The glycemic index (GI) shows how many grams of sugar, or glucose, are included in food. For example, if milk is between 15 and 30 on the GI, then milk contains between 15 and 30 g of glucose per serving.

_____ 6. Nutrients can be essential nutrients, meaning the body cannot manufacture them from other substances. As a result, they must be supplied from foods, or nonessential nutrients, which means the body does not need them, but will benefit from them.

_____ 7. Body composition is a calculated measurement using a person's weight and height to generally indicate the amount of body fat of a person.

_____ 8. The most common route for enteral nutrition involves inserting a tube through the nose and down the esophagus.

_____ 9. Water accounts for over 85% of a person's body weight.

_____ 10. In the United States, the Occupational Safety and Health Administration (OSHA) and the U.S. Department of Agriculture (USDA) mandate which foods must include the Nutrition Facts label, and set the guidelines for the information on the label.

CONTENT INSTRUCTION

Research

Find the Nutrition Facts labels on six different food items at home or in a grocery store. Record the food name or type, and the information found on the Nutrition Facts labels. Create a document, PowerPoint presentation, or other visual display of the labels that does not include the type or name of the food for each label. Create a separate visual display of the foods from which you obtained the label information. Ask your classmates to guess which food goes with each label. Record the results, and then share the correct information. Answer the questions that follow the table.

FOOD	NUMBER OF CORRECT GUESSES	NUMBER OF INCORRECT GUESSES

1. Which food/label combination was identified correctly most frequently?

_____

2. Which was identified correctly least frequently?

_____

3. Why do you think it was easier to match the Nutrition Facts labels to some foods than others?

_____

_____

_____

_____

Vitamins and Minerals

Using the chapter and other sources, fill in the missing information.

VITAMIN OR MINERAL	FUNCTIONS	FOOD SOURCES	DEFICIENCY
	Blood formation; maintain nerve tissue; metabolism of iron		Pernicious anemia; sores on mouth; loss of coordination
		Whole grain cereals, seafood, nuts, legumes, green vegetables, milk, tea, bananas	Tremors; foot cramps; convulsions; irregular heart
			Rickets, bruising, scurvy, slow healing
Vitamin B$_2$ (riboflavin)	Produce energy; healthy skin, eyes; clear vision		
			Goiter; cretinism
Vitamin B$_3$ (pantothenic acid)			Fatigue; cramps; respiratory infection; burning feet

PERFORMANCE APPLICATIONS

24-Hour Recall

Equipment and Supplies

Paper and pencil or computer

Directions

1. Choose a partner to interview for a 24-hour recall of food consumption. Use the table in Case Study 28-2 as a guide. Record the information, and then switch roles.

TIME	FOOD

Drawing Conclusions

1. Was it harder or easier than you anticipated to recall your food consumption over the last 24 hours? Why?

_____

_____

_____

_____

_____

2. Do you think a 24-hour recall or a food diary would provide a more accurate assessment of food intake? Why?

_____

_____

_____

_____

_____

_____

_____

3. Why do you think one method of assessing intake might be used over another?

_____

_____

_____

_____

_____

_____

CRITICAL THINKING

1. Review Table 28-7, Therapeutic Diets, in the textbook. Excluding the regular diet, which one do you think would be most difficult to adhere to? Why?

_____

_____

_____

_____

_____

2. Every culture in the world has rituals and practices that surround food. What are some that your culture observes? Think broadly; in this context, culture can be related to age, religion, family, and any other number of affiliations.

_____

_____

_____

_____

_____

_____

_____

_____

_____

_____

29 Emergency Medical Technicians and Paramedics

CAREERS

Careers, Duties, and Credentials

Using the chapter and other sources, fill in the missing information.

CAREER TITLE	EDUCATION	DESCRIPTION OF JOB DUTIES	LICENSURE	CREDENTIALS
Advanced emergency medical technician		Responds to medical emergencies, gives immediate care, inserts IV lines, provides medication, transports patients to health care facilities		
Emergency medical responder				
Paramedic		Provides advanced life support		
				EMT, NREMT

Education Costs and Earnings Potential

Using the Internet, research the educational cost of a prehospital responder career and the salary that might be earned in the local area. Use the information to complete the table.

CAREER	INSTITUTION FOR EDUCATION	COST OF EDUCATION	POTENTIAL EARNINGS

Skills and Qualities

Choose a career discussed in the chapter. List three personal qualities and skills that you think are important for the job and the reason(s) why.

1. _____

2. _____

3. _____

Multiple Choice

Circle the one correct answer to each of the following questions.

1. What is the "Star of Life"?
   a. A grouping of vital points in the human body
   b. A medal awarded to emergency responders for bravery
   c. A six-pointed symbol intended to make prehospital responders nationally recognizable
   d. A diagram explaining the proper steps of CPR

2. The EMR is trained to assess and assist patients who have experienced a physical injury. What is another term for physical injury?
   a. Emesis
   b. Mottle
   c. Trauma
   d. Toxin

3. What is the purpose of an automatic external defibrillator?
   a. To restore normal rhythm of the heart
   b. To close a wound
   c. To compress a blood vessel
   d. Awaken the victim

4. EMS personnel who work with the ambulance are sometimes called
   a. preemptive nurses.
   b. prehospital personnel.
   c. preemptive clinicians.
   d. first arrivers.

5. Occupational levels for emergency responders are determined by
   a. the driver's license level of the responder.
   b. the vehicle of the responder.
   c. the length of employment of the responder.
   d. the amount of training the responder has accrued.

6. Among emergency responders, which occupational level is an emergency medical responder (EMR)?
   a. The most basic
   b. One level above the most basic
   c. One level below the most advanced
   d. The most advanced

7. According to CPR guidelines for healthcare professionals, the emergency responder should
   a. pinch the nose closed and give two slow mouth-to-mouth breaths.
   b. open all airways and give two quick mouth-to-mouth breaths.
   c. open all airways and give two slow mouth-to-mouth breaths.
   d. pinch the nose closed and give two quick mouth-to-mount breaths.

8. Emergency medical technicians respond to emergencies, give immediate care, transport the victim to the hospital, and
   a. provide primary care in rural areas.
   b. act as liaison with victim's insurance company.
   c. follow-up with physician regarding victim's status
   d. maintain the rescue vehicles and equipment.

9. Which level of emergency responder is a paramedic?
   a. The most basic level of certification
   b. One level above the most basic
   c. One level below the most advanced
   d. The highest level of certification

10. A paramedic may have to perform an endotracheal intubation. What is the purpose of this technique?
    a. To measure the pulse
    b. To open the airway
    c. To stop severe bleeding
    d. To shock the heart with electric pulses

11. What is the term for immediate care given to the victim of injury or sudden illness?
    a. Triage
    b. Tourniquet
    c. CPR
    d. First aid
12. What is shock?
    a. A sudden attack of uncontrolled muscle movements
    b. A condition of acute failure of the peripheral circulation
    c. A physical injury
    d. Rapid blood loss
13. What is the term for excessive bleeding?
    a. Trauma
    b. Laceration
    c. Hemorrhage
    d. Incision
14. Which term means *vomiting*?
    a. Emesis
    b. Edema
    c. Cephalgia
    d. Neuralgia
15. Which of the following terms means setting priorities for care of victims?
    a. Aura
    b. Patency
    c. Trauma
    d. Triage

True/False

Read the following statements and write "T" for true or "F" for false in the blanks provided. If a statement is false, correct the statement to make it true.

_____ 1. An emergency medical responder, as described by the NHTSA model, is the equivalent of the NREMT certification level.

_____ 2. Paramedics are trained to administer pharmaceuticals and perform invasive procedures such as endotracheal intubations, as well as all the duties of other emergency medical personnel.

_____ 3. Open fractures break the skin, exposing the bone.

_____ 4. Hypothermia is an abnormal lowering of body temperature resulting from exposure to extreme cold.

_____ 5. EMS personnel may need to declare a mass casualty incident (MCI), where local resources are overwhelmed by the number of patients needing treatment.

_____ 6. If a patient suffers a puncture wound, the area of the injury is described as *mottled*.

_____ 7. Blood from arteries, or arterial bleeding, is bright red, whereas venous blood is darker in color.

_____ 8. Alex twisted her ankle and experienced rapid swelling of the area almost immediately. It is painful when she moves or puts pressure it. Her doctor said she injured the ligaments in her ankle. Given this information, Alex has sprained her ankle.

_____ 9. If a third-degree burn is sustained, clothing should try to be removed if possible.

_____ 10. Ice placed on an insect or snake bite will serve to speed up the poison's circulation from the area.

_____ 11. If a patient has an object penetrating their eye, first responders should not attempt to remove it.

CONTENT INSTRUCTION

Understanding the Concepts

First-aid training teaches treatment of wounds, poisoning, burns, shock, fractures, temperature alterations, illness caused by medical conditions, and other injuries. Define the conditions listed, indicate a possible cause (or causes), and describe the signs and symptoms for each.

1. Hypothermia

_____

_____

_____

_____

_____

2. Incision

_____

_____

_____

3. First-degree burn

_____

_____

_____

_____

4. Cerebrovascular accident (CVA)

_____

_____

_____

_____

_____

5. Poisoning

_____

_____

_____

_____

_____

PERFORMANCE APPLICATIONS

Pulse Point Identification

Label the pulse points in Figure 29-1.

A. _____

B. _____

C. _____

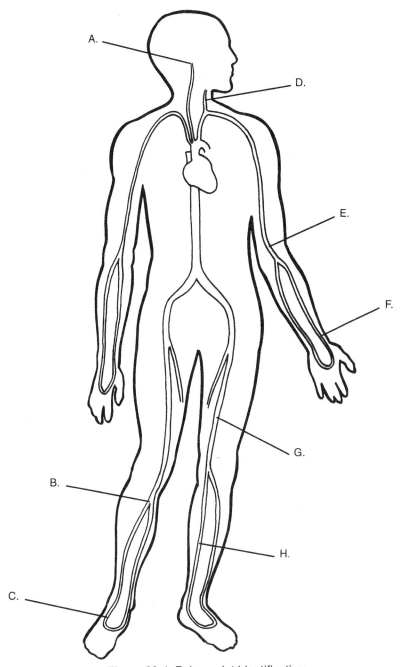

Figure 29-1 Pulse point identification.

D. _____

E. _____

F. _____

G. _____

H. _____

Casualty Simulation

Read all of the directions before beginning this activity. Laboratory activities should be completed under the supervision of a qualified professional only.

Equipment and Supplies

Paper and pencil to record evaluations
Pillows
Sheets

Directions

1. Choose a partner to role play one of the casualty simulations.
2. Choose a third person to act as the victim.
3. Consult with your partner for 3 minutes about the situation before beginning the role play.
4. Other members of the class may act as observers and evaluate the care given to the victim, using Figure 29-2.
5. Switch roles to complete the simulations.

```
EVALUATION SCALE FOR CASUALTY SIMULATION

Communicates effectively with victim                  ____/ 10 points
Communicates effectively with partner                 ____/ 5 points
Volunteers pertinent information about assessment
   and first aid treatment                            ____/ 5 points
Assesses victim for known and unknown injuries        ____/ 10 points
Correctly treats injuries                             ____/ 10 points
Gives first aid care quickly                          ____/ 5 points
Uses safety measures to protect victim and selves     ____/ 5 points
TOTAL TEAM SCORE:                                     ____/ 50 points
```

Figure 29-2

Casualty Simulation Victims

Situation 1

Your victim was working on a power pole and touched a live wire while unsuccessfully trying to break a fall. The fall was approximately 20 feet. His right hand has a third-degree burn diagonally across the palm from contact with the wire. He also has some first- and second-degree burns around the area of the third-degree burn. The victim is responsive and complaining of severe pain in his lower right arm.

Situation 2

Your victim was kicked in the chest by a horse. You find her sitting against a fence post. She is dazed and confused but responsive. She is complaining of numbness and a tingling sensation in her left arm. You can see that the left arm is displaced in a downward direction from a break in the left clavicle.

Situation 3

Your victim was running up the bleachers at school and slipped. He fell down the bleachers to the concrete below. He has a compound fracture of the left femur with moderate bleeding. He is responsive and complains of difficulty breathing.

Situation 4

Your victim is a student in a chemistry class. He knocked over a gas burner and some flammable liquid chemicals. The burning liquid ignited his shirt and jeans. The teacher pushed the student under the shower and put out the fire with water. The victim has first- and second-degree burns on his chest and both upper legs. He is pacing around the room and screaming that the pain is unbearable.

Situation 5

Your victim was injured in a car accident. She has a fractured jaw and a closed fracture of the right lower arm. She is responsive but confused.

Situation 6

Your victim had an accident while riding an all-terrain vehicle in the desert. You do not know how long he was in the desert after the accident. His breathing is rapid and shallow. His pulse is very fast. He is not responsive. His skin is hot and dry to the touch. A bruise is visible on his left upper arm, and the bone looks out of place in that area.

Drawing Conclusions

1. What first aid consideration must be made for all of the victims?

   _____

   _____

   _____

2. For each of the emergency situations described, list one measure that might have been used to prevent the injury.

   Situation 1: _____

   _____

   Situation 2: _____

   _____

   Situation 3: _____

   _____

   Situation 4: _____

   _____

   Situation 5: _____

   _____

   Situation 6: _____

   _____

CRITICAL THINKING

1. Good Samaritan laws or acts vary from state to state but usually protect any person from liability during rescues that are made out of kindness and without compensation. In some states, the Good Samaritan laws apply only to medically trained rescuers.
   Do you think Good Samaritan laws should apply to all bystanders, or be restricted to medically trained rescuers? Why?

   _____

   _____

   _____

   _____

   _____

   _____

   _____

Chapter **29** Emergency Medical Technicians and Paramedics

2. Outdoor enthusiasts and adventure seekers may encounter emergencies that require special assistance, sometimes in the form of search and rescue services. Search and rescue services are broadly defined as the search for and provision of aid to people who are in distress or imminent danger. Search and rescue is a public service in most places. However, some states charge for the service. Do you think states should charge for the service? Why or why not?

_____

_____

_____

_____

_____

_____

_____

30 Health Information Professionals

CAREERS

Careers, Duties, and Credentials

Using the chapter and other sources, fill in the missing information.

CAREER TITLE	EDUCATION	DESCRIPTION OF JOB DUTIES	LICENSURE	CREDENTIALS
Health informatician			None	
	Bachelor's degree from CAHIIM-accredited school			RHIA
			None	CMM, CMOM, CPPM, CMPE, FACMPE, ACMPE
			None	RHIT
Health services administrator				Various possibilities depending on area of specialization

Education Costs and Earnings Potential

Using the Internet, research the educational cost of one health information professional career and the salary that might be earned in the local area. Use the information to complete the table.

CAREER	INSTITUTION FOR EDUCATION	COST OF EDUCATION	POTENTIAL EARNINGS

Skills and Qualities

Choose a career discussed in the chapter. List three personal qualities and skills that you think are important for the job and the reason(s) why.

1. _____

_____

_____

_____

241

2. _____

_____

_____

_____

3. _____

_____

_____

_____

Exploring Career Opportunities

Many professional associations list career opportunities on their websites. Using one of the professional association links at the end of Chapter 30 in the textbook, search for job openings and locate the information requested below.

1. What professional association website did you choose?

_____

2. How did you find job openings on that site?

_____

_____

_____

_____

3. Choose a posted job opening to explore. What is the job title? Where is it located?

_____

_____

_____

_____

4. What are the requirements for the job? What is the compensation and/or other benefits, if listed?

_____

_____

_____

_____

_____

5. Discuss whether this job appeals to you. Why or why not?

_____

_____

_____

_____

_____

Multiple Choice

Circle the one correct answer to each of the following questions.

1. After data are collected and _____, it becomes useful information.
   a. acknowledged
   b. analyzed
   c. computerized
   d. manipulated

2. What is the correct flow of data analytics?
   a. Information → Data → Knowledge
   b. Data → Information → Knowledge
   c. Knowledge → Data → Information
   d. Data → Knowledge → Information

3. A health information management (HIM) professional is collecting statistics about the number of patients who have undergone a CABG, a type of heart surgery, at the hospital in the past year. From where does he obtain this data?
   a. Patient health records
   b. Patient surveys
   c. Physician surveys
   d. Published CDC reports

4. Which is a data element that would **not** be considered *demographic data?*
   a. Patient's phone number
   b. Patient's address
   c. Patient's race or ethnicity
   d. Patient's most recent diagnosis

5. What is the name of the legislation, signed by Congress in 1996, that addresses privacy and security within the healthcare environment?
   a. The Health Insurance Medicaid Extension Act
   b. The Health Insurance Portability and Accountability Act
   c. The Health Information Protection and Accessibility Act
   d. The Healthcare Information Privacy Act

6. RHITs may act as a _____ in multiple specialties acting where they compile and maintain data for research and public health.
   a. medical secretary
   b. medical scribe
   c. registrar
   d. transcriptionist

7. A(n) _____ degree from a CAHIIM-accredited HIM program is required to work as a Registered Health Information Administrator (RHIA).
   a. associate
   b. bachelor's
   c. master's
   d. doctoral

8. Benjamin has been taking courses online in his spare time to earn the Certified Physician Practice Manager (CPPM) credential from the AAPC. In which healthcare setting would his new credential be most useful?
   a. A large teaching hospital
   b. A smaller regional hospital
   c. A nursing home
   d. A physician's office

9. When is a discharge summary generated?
   a. Before patient admission
   b. During surgery
   c. Just before the patient leaves the facility
   d. After the patient leaves the facility

10. What is the name of the document that explains the plan for treatment, such as possible risks and any alternative treatments?
    a. Informed consent
    b. Medical record
    c. Terms of treatment
    d. HIPAA

11. What is the purpose of documenting medical necessity?
    a. To record the need for treatment
    b. To explain alternative treatments
    c. To refer the patient to a specialist
    d. To order a test, such as labs or imaging

12. The SOAP format is a way clinicians document clinical patient information. What does SOAP stand for?
    a. Subject, observation, approach, produce
    b. Sustain, observe, abstract, present
    c. Subjective, objective, assessment, plan
    d. Separate, observe, apply, plan

13. What does *authentication* throughout a patient's medical record signify?
    a. Services rendered by provider
    b. Acknowledgment of provider
    c. Correct data
    d. Provider responsibility

14. Who or what is responsible for maintaining and securing a patient's health record?
    a. The patient
    b. The provider, hospital, or clinic
    c. The government
    d. The patient's family

15. What information is in the *master patient index*?
    a. List of all medical supply vendors
    b. List of services provided
    c. List of physicians on staff
    d. List of all patients seen and serviced

16. Which is an example of using the health record to support *compliance*?
    a. A patient's lawyer reviews the health record to see how the physician recorded the diagnosis.
    b. The Joint Commission reviews health records to review the care offered to patients.
    c. A researcher aggregates health record data to examine how well a treatment is working.
    d. A specialist reviews the record to see what treatments the patient has already tried.

17. The community clinic is noticing an increase in new cases of chlamydia. What is the medical term for "new cases of disease?"
    a. Statistic
    b. Morbidity
    c. Mortality
    d. Incidence

18. The HIM function of summarizing all the information in a health record is called
    a. abstracting.
    b. conveying.
    c. presenting.
    d. analyzing.

19. What is the term for a total picture of the patient's health and the services delivered over time, regardless of setting and provider?
    a. Master patient index
    b. Patient table
    c. Longitudinal record
    d. Patient registry

20. Risk management is the coordination of efforts inside a healthcare organization to prevent and control PCEs. What does PCE stand for?
    a. Partially criminal employees
    b. Primary care expenses
    c. Poorly constructed entities
    d. Potentially compensable events

Matching

Match each numbered term with its best definition.

Term	Definition
_____ 1. Coding	A. Speaking words to be written by another person; may be recorded
_____ 2. Compliance	B. To make a written copy of dictated or recorded matter
_____ 3. Deficiency	C. Assignment of alphanumerical codes to diagnoses and procedures
_____ 4. Dictation	D. A command to a database to retrieve desired data or reports
_____ 5. Transcription	E. An element missing from a health record
_____ 6. Query	F. Adherence to standards

CONTENT INSTRUCTION

Sorting

Assign each example of data with the letter reflecting its type.

Types of Data	
C	Clinical
D	Demographic
F	Financial
L	Legal

Examples of Data

1. Name	_____
2. Patient's employer	_____
3. Patient history	_____
4. Mailing address	_____
5. Operative report	_____
6. Consent to treatment	_____

(Continued)

7. Social Security number	_____
8. Notice of Privacy Practices	_____
9. Imaging report	_____
10. Date of birth	_____
11. Guarantor	_____
12. Nursing notes	_____
13. Advance directives	_____
14. Primary payer	_____
15. Medical proxy	_____

Privacy and Security of Health Information

The Health Insurance Portability and Accountability Act (HIPAA) of 1996 is the primary legislation protecting individuals' private information. HIPAA limits the communication of all protected health information (PHI), defined as health data that can be identified with an individual. This means that any information concerning the patient's health status connected to, for example, the patient's name, address, telephone number, date of birth, or other identification must be kept strictly confidential.

The creation and implementation of HIPAA required considerable work for many parties, including legislators, enforcement agencies, providers, and health information professionals. Using the Internet and other sources, research the following questions.

1. How was private health information protected prior to HIPAA?

_____

_____

_____

_____

2. What were some of the problems that occurred when private health information was not protected under HIPAA?

_____

_____

_____

_____

_____

_____

_____

_____

3. Do you think the use of electronic health records has made it more or less difficult to access health information? Why or why not?

_____

_____

_____

_____

_____

_____

_____

_____

_____

_____

Risk Management

After reading the scenario, assign each example of a potentially compensable event (PCE) with the letters reflecting its type of risk, according to the table. Indicate why the situation poses that risk.

Type of Risk	
PS	Patient safety
MFR	Mandatory federal regulations
PME	Potential medical errors
EFP	Existing and future policy
L	Legislation impacting the healthcare field

You are a newly hired health services administrator at a small long-term care facility. The previous health services administrator, Judith Penrod, had been in ill health and frequently absent for some time before retiring. You find that quite a few risk management issues need to be addressed.

1. A maintenance order indicates that three beds have faulty side rails; the rails cannot be raised on two of the beds and won't lower on the third. When you check with the maintenance crew, you learn that these beds were never fixed. Not only that, but there are also patients currently in all three.

   Type of risk: _____

   Why?

   _____

   _____

   _____

2. On your second day, you make rounds of several units. You overhear one of the aides talking to a visitor about Mrs Lawrence, a resident. The aide tells the visitor, who lives next door to Mrs Lawrence's daughter in town, "Make sure you tell Mrs. Lawrence's daughter about how high her mother's sugar's been running. She needs to get in here and give her mother a talking to about staying away from the sweets!"

Type of risk: _____

Why:

_____

_____

_____

_____

3. When you get home one evening during your second week on the job, you decide to do some "light reading" of a professional newsletter. The feature article is about potential changes to Medicaid reimbursement, specifically for residents of long-term care facilities. The majority of the residents in your facility are on Medicaid. It looks like considerably more documentation might be required for continued reimbursement at the same level if lawmakers agree to move the bill forward.

Type of risk: _____

Why:

_____

_____

_____

_____

4. The nurses and aides on a particular unit have worked at the facility longer than anyone else. They are, as a whole, kind and dedicated to the patients in their care. They are also very busy. You notice that blood samples will sometimes sit overnight before being sent to the laboratory. This allows for potential degradation of the sample, which could then return inaccurate results.

Type of risk: _____

Why:

_____

_____

5. The facility is just beginning to use electronic health records. The paper records are still housed in large filing cabinets on each unit. Although you're happy to see that the use of EHR being implemented, you are not sure what to do with all the paper records after the use of EHR has been established.

Type of risk: _____

Why:

_____

_____

_____

_____

PERFORMANCE INSTRUCTION

Registries

Health data is frequently abstracted for research and quality measures. The Centers for Disease Control and Prevention maintain statistics based on the data gathered by National Program of Cancer Registries. Visit the CDC at https://www.cdc.gov/cancer/npcr/index.htm. Watch the video "Cancer Registries: Measuring Progress. Targeting Action," then answer the following questions.

1. What five questions does the registry data enable the CDC to answer?

   a. _____

   b. _____

   c. _____

   d. _____

   e. _____

2. What does the CDC use registry data for?

   a. _____

   b. _____

   c. _____

3. _____

4. Who can view the registry data on the CDC website?_____

On the same website, use the link under Contact a Local Registry to view data presentation about the incidence of cancer in the United States. Click on three states to compare data under the State-specific Cancer Statistics heading. Note that you are able to view the data in a table or chart visualization.

1. Which three states did you research?

   _____

2. For each state, what were the top three cancers by rate of new cancer cases?

   _____

   _____

   _____

3. For each state, what were the top three cancers by rate of cancer deaths?

   _____

   _____

   _____

4. Did you prefer the table or chart data visualization?

   _____

Graphing Practice

Gather and chart the following data.

- Height of each student in class in centimeters: chart the data as a line graph using the height as the independent variable and the number of students of that height as the dependent variable. See Skill List 30-2 and 30-3 in the textbook for instructions on creating graphs.
- Age of each student in months: chart the data as a bar graph using the age as the independent variable and the number of students of that age as the dependent variable.
- Student zip code: choose a charting method that could be used to show the percentage of students from each zip code.

Questions

1. Using the graph, what can you conclude, if anything, about the height of people in your class?

   _____

   _____

   _____

249

2. Using the graph, what can you conclude, if anything, about the age of people in your class?

_____

_____

_____

3. Using the graph, what can you conclude, if anything, about the places where students live?

_____

_____

_____

CRITICAL THINKING

Ownership of the health record is an interesting topic and the cause of some confusion among patients and even among those within the healthcare industry. There is no consensus on who owns health records, and both federal and state laws are unclear or inconsistent. However, the common thinking is that the patient owns the information in the record, but not the medium in which the information is kept.

This has led to inconsistent policies and implementation regarding release of information requests. Oftentimes, healthcare information must be shared between healthcare facilities. This sharing of information occurs through a health information exchange (HIE) that allows different computers systems to access each other's data via interoperable technologies. However, one of the biggest hurdles to interoperability comes from the providers and EHR vendors themselves, who are sometimes reluctant to share patient information. As a business, a provider would prefer a patient choose to obtain services within its system rather than seek treatment elsewhere; a software vendor would prefer a provider buy and use its software to communicate with another health provider rather than make its data easily available across platforms. The so-called "information blocking" practices include ignoring patient requests for information, insisting on using a fax machine instead of the EHR, or charging outside providers high fees to use a secure connection.

1. Who do you think should own the medical record? Why?

_____

_____

_____

_____

_____

2. In your opinion, should EHR developers be required to make their technologies interoperable? Why or why not?

_____

_____

_____

_____

_____

3. What do you think is a reasonable policy for a healthcare provider or facility to implement regarding patients' requests for release of information? For example, how long should a patient wait for release of medical records? What should the provider or facility charge the patient to obtain his or her medical records? Should that amount be prorated based on the number of pages provided? Should the records be released only in one format (i.e., electronic or paper)? Provide a rationale for your policy.

_____

_____

_____

_____

_____

_____

_____

_____

_____

_____

_____

_____

_____

_____

_____

_____

31 Health Insurance Professionals

Careers, Duties, and Credentials

Using the chapter and other sources, fill in the missing information.

CAREER TITLE	EDUCATION	DESCRIPTION OF JOB DUTIES	LICENSURE	CREDENTIALS
Claims assistant professional			Some states require licensure	
Medical biller/claims processor				CPB, CBCS, CMRS, CMBS, CMIS
	Diploma program or associate degree	Review clinical documentation using the patient's health records and convert the diagnosis, tests, procedures, and treatments to standardized codes		CPC, CIC, COC, CPC-H, CPMA, CRC, CCS, CCS-P, CCA, HIM, RHIA, RHIT, CHP, CHPS, CHS, CDIP, BCSC, CMC, CMCS
Medical auditor			No licensure, but some states require national certification as medical coder and/or professional medical auditor	

Education Costs and Earnings Potential

Using the Internet, research the educational cost of one health insurance professional career and the salary that might be earned in the local area. Use the information to complete the table.

CAREER	INSTITUTION FOR EDUCATION	COST OF EDUCATION	POTENTIAL EARNINGS

Skills and Qualities

Choose a career discussed in the chapter. List three personal qualities and skills that you think are important for the job and the reason(s) why.

1. _____

_____

_____

_____

2. _____

_____

_____

_____

3. _____

_____

_____

_____

Exploring Career Opportunities

Many professional associations list career opportunities on their websites. Using one of the professional association links at the end of Chapter 31 in the textbook, search for job openings and locate the information requested below.

1. What professional association website did you choose?

_____

2. How did you find job openings on that site?

_____

_____

_____

3. Choose a posted job opening to explore. What is the job title? Where is it located?

_____

_____

_____

_____

4. What are the requirements for the job? What is the compensation and/or other benefits, if listed?

_____

_____

_____

_____

_____

5. Discuss whether this job appeals to you. Why or why not?

_____

_____

_____

_____

_____

_____

Multiple Choice

Circle the one correct answer to each of the following questions.

1. The insurance company, Aetna, is determining whether or not to pay for all or some of the claim submitted by Mr Wilson's provider. What is this process called?
   a. Medical necessity
   b. Explanation of benefits
   c. Reimbursement
   d. Adjudication

2. Dr Moore's office did a very thorough job on the claim it submitted, including accurate coding. It has all the necessary information and will likely be approved because it is a(n)
   a. accurate claim.
   b. authentic claim.
   c. clean claim.
   d. correct claim.

3. What is the explanation of benefits (EOB)?
   a. A patient rights form given to a patient upon admission to the hospital
   b. A document from the insurer with details on what was covered and why
   c. A form sent to the provider about compensation
   d. An annual statement outlining insurance coverage

4. Which is **not** an example of a *third-party payer*?
   a. The patient
   b. An insurance company
   c. Medicare
   d. Medicaid

5. Which is **not** a duty of a medical biller?
   a. Coding
   b. Preparing claims
   c. Taking vital signs of patients
   d. Submitting claims

6. Andrews's sister, Claire, is a medical biller for a large hospital in California. Claire likes her job and mentions that the hospital is "desperate" for medical billers and claims processors. Andrew thinks he might find this line of work rewarding. Since graduating from high school, he has had a few years of work experience as a server at a restaurant. What additional education or training should he pursue, at a minimum?
   a. Associate degree
   b. Master's degree and supervised internship
   c. Bachelor's degree
   d. Training program and certification

7. The job of a claims assistant professional is _____, meaning no prior work experience is necessary.
   a. non-exempt
   b. part-time
   c. entry-level
   d. managerial

8. Which credential is offered by the American Health Information Management Association (AHIMA)?
   a. Certified Professional Coder (CPC)
   b. Certified Medical Coder (CMC)
   c. Certified Coding Specialist (CCS)
   d. Certified Medical Coding Specialist (CMCS)

9. In the last 20 years, _____ has been available to help with medical coding and reduce errors.
   a. complete and accurate coding (CAC) software
   b. computer-assisted coding (CAC) software
   c. corrective assurance coding (CAC) software
   d. corrective accuracy of coding (CAC) software

10. What is the function of *natural language processing (NLP)*?
    a. To automatically generate medical codes by analyzing keywords and phrases in a patient's medical record
    b. To transfer dictated provider notes into transcribed, computerized record entries
    c. To scan a patient's electronic health record (EHR) for errors and automatically correcting them
    d. To interpret the words of non-English-speaking patients
11. If a physical therapist's office submits a claim for a 1-hour therapy session with detailed patient education, when in fact the session took much less time and no patient education was offered, the provider has committed
    a. malpractice
    b. battery
    c. laterality
    d. fraud
12. Which code set is used to record the patient's diagnosis in all settings?
    a. Current Procedural Terminology (CPT)
    b. ICD-10-PCS
    c. ICD-10-CM
    d. HCPCS
13. The pain management clinic uses a computer program to automate claims from preparation to tracking reimbursement. What is the name of this software?
    a. Practice management program
    b. Process management program
    c. Process module program
    d. Proven method program
14. What is the likely result when a medical biller at a physician's office submits a claim with a coding error?
    a. The provider will be fined.
    b. The medical biller will be brought to court.
    c. The claim will be denied.
    d. The provider will lose his or her license.
15. What is the meaning of the term upcoding?
    a. Advanced, quicker method of coding
    b. Using both ICD and PCS codes to represent the treatment(s) provided
    c. Assigning an inaccurate billing code in order to increase reimbursement
    d. Using Level II HCPCS codes rather than Level I HCPCS codes for simplicity and quicker reimbursement
16. In what year did the United States begin using the 10th revision of the International Classification of Diseases, ICD-10-CM?
    a. 1985
    b. 1962
    c. 2021
    d. 2015
17. The increase in total codes from ICD-9-CM to ICD-10-CM is about 56,000, due largely to the inclusion of *laterality*, which means
    a. the difference in how a condition presents or what approach was taken to treat the condition.
    b. the labeling of certain areas of the body, such as head, neck, trunk, and limbs.
    c. the methods used for a procedure, such as moving the instrument or machine in a sideways direction.
    d. the indication of the side of the body on which a procedure was performed, or which was affected by a condition.
18. Coding to the highest degree of _____ should be used to ensure clean claims.
    a. complexity
    b. simplicity
    c. specificity
    d. privacy
19. What might a capital or lowercase X ("X" or "x") be used for in ICD-10-CM coding?
    a. A placeholder
    b. A modifier
    c. A subset character
    d. An essential modifier

20. What is the first step of the medical billing cycle?
    a. The provider sees the patient
    b. A prospective patient is scheduled or preregistered
    c. The visit is coded
    d. The claim is prepared and submitted

True/False

Read the following statements and write "T" for true or "F" for false in the blanks provided. If a statement is false, correct the statement to make it true.

_____ 1. An eponym is a name of a drug or a disease based on or derived from a person's name.

_____ 2. ICD-10-PCS codes are used to describe procedures performed in outpatient settings.

_____ 3. Category I CPT codes are alphanumeric.

_____ 4. During patient checkout, the physician or provider is responsible for calculating balances, copays, coinsurance, as well as any new charges for the visit that just occurred.

_____ 5. Simple errors are often the cause of claim rejection.

_____ 6. The first step of the coding process is locating the code in the Tabular List of Diseases and Injuries.

_____ 7. Using both the Alphabetic Index and Tabular List is important when assigning a code.

_____ 8. Before submitting a code, it is important to check modifiers for the procedure or service in order to reach the highest level of specificity.

_____ 9. Immediately after a patient's appointment, detailed demographic and medical information is collected.

_____ 10. Another name for an encounter form is *superbill*.

CONTENT INSTRUCTION

Fill in the Blank

Fill in each of the spaces provided with the missing word or words that complete the sentence.

1. The health insurance claims process is an interaction between the healthcare provider and the _____, and usually takes several days to several months to complete.

2. For a claim submission to be reimbursed, it must meet the _____ necessity criteria.

3. A(n) _____ is a document prepared by the insurance carrier that gives details on how the claim was adjudicated.

4. _____ is the process of determining how a claim should be paid or denied after comparing it to the coverage outlined in the healthcare policy.

5. Medical health insurance claims submitted on paper use a standardized form called the

   _____

6. The electronic version of the standardized form used to submit medical health insurance claims is called the

   _____.

7. ICD-10 codes are divided into two systems: _____ and

   _____

8. The cardinal rule of coding is never to code from the _____ alone.

9. The _____ of the ICD-10-CM coding manual is divided into chapters based on body system/anatomic site, or condition/etiology.

10. If a code requires a 7th character is not 6 characters long, _____ must be used to fill in the empty characters.

Understanding the Concepts

Answer the following questions in your own words.

1. Jill Bradford saw her primary care provider, Dr Simonelli, because she has been experiencing nausea and indigestion. Dr Simonelli takes a history and orders tests. Jonathan, the medical billing specialist and coder in Dr Simonelli's office, knows not to use specific diagnosis codes until the test results come back and Dr Simonelli has established a diagnosis. What does Jonathan do instead?

   _____

   _____

2. Leonard Opelika visited an urgent care center because he was having chest pain. The physician there took a history, performed a general physical examination, and had his medical assistant do an electrocardiogram. The claim submitted to Leonard's insurance company includes charges for the history and physical exam, the electrocardiogram, and echocardiography. What is wrong with this claim?

_____

3. Dr Lorien's practice is in a small rural town in New Mexico. It's just Dr Lorien and her assistant, Pamela, working there. They are "old school," still making house calls as needed, keeping physical patient records, and hiring a book-keeper one day a week to log payments and accounts receivable. Dr Lorien doesn't even accept credit card payments! What form does Dr Lorien's practice most likely use to bill Medicare?

_____

PERFORMANCE INSTRUCTION

For each step in Box 31-9, Keys to Successful Claims Processing, in the textbook, indicate whether the step is performed before or after the patient's encounter with the healthcare provider. Then, list one or more action(s) you could take to make sure you followed the step correctly. The first step, "Collect and verify patient information," is completed as an example.

Step	Before/After Encounter	Action to Take
Collect and verify patient information	Before	Ask the patient to spell their name; double check insurance information.
Obtain necessary preauthorization and/or precertification		
Ensure proper documentation		
Proofread claims to avoid errors		
Submit a clean claim		

CRITICAL THINKING

1. Many of the careers discussed in this chapter require only a high school diploma or equivalent for entry. For example, a medical claims processor requires only a high school diploma or equivalent, and on-the-job training or completion of voluntary certification. Based on what you have learned about other healthcare professions, is the education require-ment for health insurance professionals what you expected it would be? Why or why not?

_____

_____

_____

_____

2. Do you think setting minimum standards for training and education for health insurance professionals would be beneficial? Why or why not?

_____

_____

_____

_____

_____

_____

_____

_____

32 Dental Professionals

Careers, Duties, and Credentials

Using the chapter and other sources, fill in the missing information.

CAREER TITLE	EDUCATION	DESCRIPTION OF JOB DUTIES	LICENSURE	CREDENTIALS
Dental laboratory technician			None	
	Bachelor's degree, or a combination of experience and associate's degree		Licensed by state	RDH
		Examines patients, diagnoses disease and other problems, directs care, and provides treatment		
		Considerable variation in responsibilities, but might include answering phones, passing equipment to the dentist during procedures, and maintaining infection control		Varied certifications through DANB

Education Costs and Earnings Potential

Using the Internet, research the educational cost of a dental professional career and the salary that might be earned in the local area. Use the information to complete the table.

CAREER	INSTITUTION FOR EDUCATION	COST OF EDUCATION	POTENTIAL EARNINGS

Skills and Qualities

Choose a career discussed in the chapter. List three personal qualities and skills that you think are important for the job and the reason(s) why.

1. _____

2. _____

3. _____

Multiple Choice

Circle the one correct answer to each of the following questions.

1. What is the term for missing teeth?
   a. Gingivitis
   b. Halitosis
   c. Malocclusion
   d. Edentulism

2. What is another term for cavities?
   a. Dental caries
   b. Amalgam
   c. Alveoli
   d. Crown

3. Dentists are skilled in radiology, meaning they are capable of dealing with
   a. electronic pulse anesthesia.
   b. laboratory tests.
   c. braces.
   d. X-rays.

4. Sally works in a dental office and has many duties from answering the phone to assessing vital signs and exposing X-rays. She also makes sure to take and record full dental histories. What is Sally's position?
   a. Dentist
   b. Dental assistant
   c. Dental hygienist
   d. Dental laboratory technician

5. Which dental specialty treats disease inside the tooth?
   a. Pedodontics
   b. Prosthodontics
   c. Endodontics
   d. Periodontics

6. Kayleigh is being fitted for braces this afternoon. She is seeing Dr Smith, who is a dentist practicing which specialty?
   a. Pedodontics
   b. Orthodontics
   c. Endodontics
   d. Prosthodontics

7. Which dental specialty aims to prevent disease and decay in the teeth of children?
   a. Periodontics
   b. Public health dentistry
   c. Pedodontics
   d. Prosthodontics

8. Amanda wants to be a dental hygienist and is preparing for her future. What level of education must Amanda reach?
   a. High-school diploma
   b. Associate degree
   c. Bachelor's degree
   d. High-school diploma and certificate in Dental Hygiene

9. Which of the following tasks might a dental lab technician do?
   a. Removing calculus from a patient's teeth and gums
   b. Root planning
   c. Creating protheses, such as bridges, dentures, and crowns
   d. Examining the oral cavity for issues

10. The American Dental Association recommends the following preventative care:
    a. Brushing once per day, flossing once per week.
    b. Brushing once per day, flossing twice per week.
    c. Brushing twice per day, flossing once per day.
    d. Brushing twice per day, flossing once per week.

11. Scaling is a function performed by dental hygienists. It involves
    a. polishing of the teeth.
    b. measuring of crowns.
    c. preparing molds.
    d. removing calculus from below the gumline.
12. Inflammation of the gums is referred to as
    a. halitosis.
    b. bruxism.
    c. gingivitis.
    d. periodontitis.
13. The longest and strongest bone of the face is the
    a. mandible.
    b. maxilla.
    c. soft palate.
    d. hard palate.
14. The teeth are located in sockets of the mandible and maxilla. What is another term for these sockets?
    a. Caries
    b. Oral cavity
    c. Edentulous
    d. Alveoli
15. The term maxilla means which part of the face?
    a. Roof of the mouth
    b. Lower jaw
    c. Cheek
    d. Upper jaw
16. At birth, the neonate has _____ tooth buds at various stages of development.
    a. 44
    b. 22
    c. 32
    d. 64
17. The _____ teeth replace the deciduous teeth at about age 12, but might not completely appear until age 20.
    a. primary
    b. interim
    c. temporary
    d. permanent
18. Which of the following types of teeth are primarily used for tearing?
    a. Incisors
    b. Molars
    c. Bicuspids
    d. Cuspids
19. Which of the following types of teeth are the largest and strongest?
    a. Molars
    b. Cuspids
    c. Bicuspids
    d. Incisors
20. The Universal System for numbering teeth counts the primary teeth using labels with letters A though:
    a. S
    b. Z
    c. B
    d. T
21. When an X-ray beam hits a dense tissue such as bone or teeth, what happens?
    a. The beam is prevented from reaching the tubehead.
    b. The tissue obstructs the beam from reaching the receptor.
    c. The beam passes through the dense tissue.
    d. The beam sensitizes the areas of the receptor behind the dense tissue.

22. What does a dosimetry badge measure?
    a. The amount of radiation to which the worker has been exposed.
    b. The amount of radiation to which the patient has been exposed.
    c. The size and shape of the patient's dentition.
    d. The amount of radiation in a single X-ray exposure.
23. Which is **not** a benefit of digital X-ray technology?
    a. Less prone to processing errors
    b. Faster to produce images
    c. Inexpensive equipment
    d. Use less radiation
24. _____ is the material used to fill caries.
    a. Amalgam
    b. Gingiva
    c. Plaster
    d. Dentition

True/False

Read the following statements and write "T" for true or "F" for false in the blanks provided. If a statement is false, correct the statement to make it true.

_____ 1. An alveolus is a localized collection of pus in a cavity formed by destruction of tissue.

_____ 2. Some states allow dental hygienists to diagnose and treat dental hygiene conditions and create treatment plans for the patient.

_____ 3. Most students entering dental school have completed a 4-year Bachelor of Science degree and anticipate earning a DDS or DMD degree in about 3–4 years.

_____ 4. Brushing removes plaque and prevents bad breath, also called bruxism.

_____ 5. The roof of the mouth is divided into two portions, the hard palate and the soft palate.

_____ 6. Periodontal disease is caused by an infection within the tooth itself.

_____ 7. Teeth are located in the mandibular and maxillary arches.

_____ 8. Tooth formation begins after the baby is born.

_____ 9. Descriptive anatomy of the tooth is called odontology.

_____ 10. The Universal System numbers the adult teeth from 1 to 16 beginning with the left maxillary third molar to the right maxillary third molar.

CONTENT INSTRUCTION

Understanding the Concepts

Using your own words, answer each question in two or three sentences.

1. Dentures are replacement prostheses for total tooth loss. What functions do they serve for the wearer? How should dentures be cared for?

_____

_____

_____

2. Describe the composition of the crown of the tooth.

_____

_____

_____

_____

3. Why are impacted or partially erupted wisdom teeth sometimes extracted?

_____

_____

_____

_____

_____

4. What are three conditions that can be visualized with dental radiographs?

_____

_____

_____

_____

_____

_____

Identifying Structures of the Oral Cavity

Write the name of the lettered structure in the appropriate space below.

A. _____   D. _____

B. _____   E. _____

C. _____   F. _____

Identifying Structures of the Tooth

Write the name of the lettered structure in the appropriate space below.

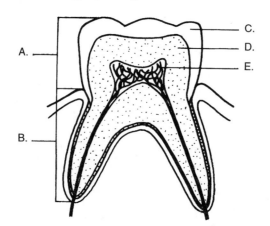

A. _____ D. _____

B. _____ E. _____

C. _____

Identifying the Teeth in the Mouth

Write the name of the lettered structure in the appropriate space below.

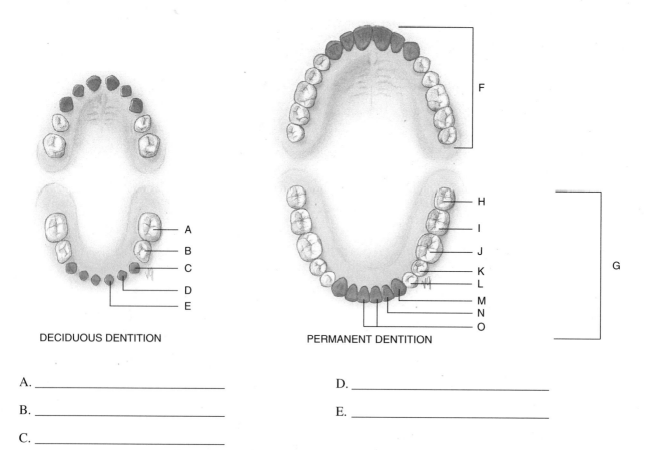

DECIDUOUS DENTITION   PERMANENT DENTITION

A. _____ D. _____

B. _____ E. _____

C. _____

Identifying Surfaces of the Teeth

Write the name of the lettered structure in the appropriate space below.

A. _____   D. _____

B. _____   E. _____

C. _____

Charting Dental Structures

Mrs Smith, a 62-year-old woman, has the dental history shown in the table.

Mrs. Smith Dental History.

TOOTH NUMBER	DENTAL STRUCTURE
1	Tooth missing
2	Amalgam restoration
3	Amalgam restoration
14	Esthetic restoration
15	Gold crown
16	Tooth missing
17	Amalgam restoration
18	Caries or decay
31	Root canal
32	Gold crown

Use Figure 32-12 of the textbook to chart the information regarding Mrs Smith's dentition on the diagram of the teeth below.

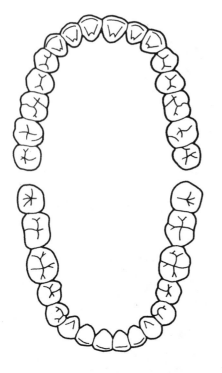
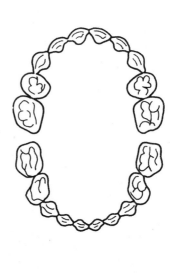

Questions

1. Why is it normal for the third molars to be missing?

_____

_____

_____

2. Why would Mrs Smith need a dental visit?

_____

_____

PERFORMANCE INSTRUCTION

Practicing Oral Hygiene

Read all of the directions before beginning this activity. Laboratory activities should be completed under the supervision of a qualified professional only.

Equipment and Supplies

Dental floss
Disclosing tablet
Mirror
Toothbrush
Toothpaste

Directions

1. Practice medical asepsis by using good handwashing technique.
2. Brush your teeth for 3 minutes using a toothbrush and toothpaste of preference.
3. Floss your teeth as instructed in the textbook.

4. Chew a disclosing tablet provided by your instructor.
5. Use a mirror to identify the areas missed during brushing and flossing.
6. Brush your teeth to remove all color remaining from the tablet.

Questions

1. Which areas of your teeth, if any, did you omit in brushing?

_____

_____

2. Why would it be more likely for a cavity to form on a tooth that is habitually missed during brushing?

_____

_____

_____

_____

_____

CRITICAL THINKING

Dental Phobia

Between 9% and 20% of Americans suffer from some degree of dental phobia, or an irrational fear of dental examination. Symptoms of this problem include anxiety and physiological changes related to stress. Some techniques have been developed to reduce the phobia related to dental appointments, including resisting the negative thoughts about the visit before seeing the dentist. It has also been demonstrated that it may be helpful for the patient to focus on taking regular breaths during the visit and to inform the dentist when fear is present. Focusing on positive thoughts, such as "I am getting good care and improving my health," also may be helpful.

1. Why do you think some people experience dental phobia?

_____

_____

_____

_____

_____

2. What other suggestions could you make to reduce the anxiety of the dental visit?

_____

_____

_____

_____

_____

_____

3. What could a health care worker do in the office to reduce the dental phobia of the patient?

_____

_____

_____

_____

_____

4. What other statements could be used to generate positive thoughts and promote concentration during the appointment?

_____

_____

_____

_____

_____

5. Why is it important to communicate the fear of a dental visit to the dentist?

_____

_____

_____

_____

_____

Dental Hygienists' Expanding Scope of Practice

Many states have scope of practice laws that allow registered dental hygienists to perform preventative treatment without the prior examination of the patient by a dentist. Some states even allow the dental hygienist to administer local anesthesia without the supervision of a dentist on the premises. A handful of states allow dental hygienists to diagnose and treat dental hygiene conditions and create dental hygiene treatment plans.

1. What are some reasons that a state may choose to expand the scope of practice for dental hygienists?

_____

_____

_____

_____

_____

2. What groups might be in favor of the expanded scope of practice of dental hygienists? Why? What groups might be opposed to the expanded scope of practice of dental hygienists? Why?

_____

_____

_____

_____

_____

_____

_____

_____

_____

_____

33 Complementary and Alternative Medicine Careers

CAREERS

Careers, Duties, and Credentials

Using the chapter and other sources, fill in the missing information.

CAREER TITLE	EDUCATION	DESCRIPTION OF JOB DUTIES	LICENSURE	CREDENTIALS
Chiropractor				
			Most states require licensure and certification	L.Ac.
		Primary care physician who performs routine medical examinations, laboratory tests, and office procedures, such as minor surgery		
Biofeedback practitioner				
	500–1000 hours of study, training, and clinical experience. Most students finish school in 1 or 2 years.	Uses skillful touch to loosen muscles and relieve pain		

Education Costs and Earnings Potential

Using the Internet, research the educational cost of one complementary and alternative medicine career and the salary that might be earned in the local area. Use the information to complete the table.

CAREER	INSTITUTION FOR EDUCATION	COST OF EDUCATION	POTENTIAL EARNINGS

Skills and Qualities

Choose a career discussed in the chapter. List three personal qualities and skills that you think are important for the job and the reason(s) why.

1. _____

2. _____

3. _____

273

KNOWLEDGE CHECK

Multiple Choice

1. What is the term that refers to the view of health that considers the entire body, as well as social and mental factors?
   a. Holistic
   b. Allopathic
   c. Orthopedics
   d. Biology

2. Prana and qi are types of
   a. biofields.
   b. reiki.
   c. massage techniques.
   d. dietary supplements.

3. What treatments are offered in homeopathy?
   a. Guided imagery
   b. Chelation
   c. Remedies
   d. Gua sha

4. What is reflexology?
   a. The practice of scraping the skin to improve blood flow
   b. Meditation and low-impact movements to facilitate movement of qi
   c. The application of pressure to areas of the foot
   d. Rubbing of the soft tissue to increase circulation and promote relaxation.

5. Which practitioner corrects misalignments of the spine?
   a. Naturopath
   b. Acupuncturist
   c. Chiropractor
   d. Biofeedback Technician

6. What is hypnotherapy?
   a. A mind-body intervention in which a patient visualizes the healing process
   b. The practice of the self-regulation using mental activity
   c. The changing of behaviors through suggestion while patient is deeply relaxed
   d. Using dance and other forms of creative expression to heal

7. Which of the following terms means an incomplete of partial dislocation?
   a. Subluxation
   b. Sublingual
   c. Chelation
   d. Cupping

8. In addition to undergraduate education, students studying to be a chiropractor must also attend an accredited chiropractic program, which is a minimum of
   a. 18 months.
   b. 4 years.
   c. 2 years.
   d. 12 months.

9. Hydrotherapy is a holistic technique involving
   a. the internal use of water, hydration.
   b. the external use of essential oils.
   c. the internal use of essential oils by way of inhalation.
   d. the external use of water.

10. Which is a brief description of acupuncture?
    a. Administering a chemical agent to aid the elimination of metals from the body
    b. Encouraging expression the dance
    c. Scraping of the skin to improve blood flow
    d. Inserting needles into the skin to change the flow of qi

11. Which technique gives the patient conscious control of involuntary reactions?
    a. Acupuncture
    b. Hypnotherapy
    c. Biofeedback
    d. Reiki

12. Mark is seeing a holistic therapist who is educating him on how to visualize his white blood cells and having him imagine they are destroying his cancer cells. What type of mind–body intervention is this?
    a. Guided imagery
    b. Meditation
    c. Expressive therapy
    d. Hypnotherapy

13. What is the best description of massage therapy?
    a. Skillfully touching to loosen muscles and relieve pain
    b. Using suggestions while patient is in a deep state of relaxation
    c. Transferring energy from the hands of the practitioner to the patient's body
    d. Strategically placing needles into the patient's skin to change the flow of qi

14. Which therapy involves using chemicals and vitamins in megadoses?
    a. Moxibustion
    b. Aromatherapy
    c. Orthomolecular therapy
    d. Reiki

15. Reiki is based on the idea that there is a universal source of energy that
    a. allows the body to perform daily activities.
    b. can influence the mood.
    c. can be removed with gemstones.
    d. allows the body to heal.

16. In acupuncture, what is a meridian?
    a. A pathway of the body through which qi flows
    b. A needle
    c. A smoldering herb
    d. A pressure area on the foot

True/False

____ 1. Therapies are considered alternative when they are used alongside of allopathic medicine.
____ 2. Homeopathy, a holistic treatment modality, is based on the concept that "like cures like."
____ 3. Since 2010, all complementary and alternative medicine practitioners are required to be licensed.
____ 4. Homeopaths cannot prescribe medication and must be careful not to diagnose disease.
____ 5. A licensed naturopathic doctor is permitted to prescribe medications and diagnose disease.
____ 6. A traditional naturopath attends a 4-year federally-accredited medical school before taking the NPLEX.
____ 7. Naturopaths view some disease processes as related to the buildup of toxins in the body.
____ 8. Biofeedback is an energy therapy.
____ 9. In depuration, the sauna is thought to cause the excretion of pollutants from the body.
____ 10. Stress dots made of liquid crystal are used in the holistic practice of acupuncture.
____ 11. Aromatherapy uses essential oils to treat diseases by having the patient inhale the substances or applying them externally on their body.

CONTENT INSTRUCTION

Describing the Domains

Describe each of the five categories or domains of complementary and alternative medicine and give examples of each.

1. Alternative medical systems

_____

_____

_____

2. Mind–body interventions

_____

_____

_____

3. Biologically based therapy

_____

_____

_____

4. Manipulative and body-based methods

_____

_____

_____

5. Energy therapy

_____

_____

_____

PERFORMANCE APPLICATION

Using Biofeedback to Measure and Control Body Reactions

Read all the instructions before beginning this activity. Laboratory activities should be completed under the supervision of a qualified professional only.

Equipment and Supplies

Liquid crystal thermal indicator (Biodot)

Directions

1. Wash and dry both hands thoroughly.
2. Apply a liquid crystal thermal indicator to the flap between the thumb and index finger on the hand that is not dominant.
3. Note the color of the Biodot in the table below.
4. Monitor the color of the Biodot throughout the rest of the day, noting the time and activity of any color change. Data collection is complete when the Biodot becomes dislodged.
5. Record the information in the table for any color change that occurs.

TIME OF READING	COLOR OF BIODOT	ACTIVITY
Initial =		

Questions

1. What type of activity was the most stressful, using the Biodot as the indicator of your stress level?

_____

_____

_____

2. Did you feel most stressed during the activity indicated to be stressful by the Biodot?

_____

_____

_____

3. What are some other factors that might influence the reading of the Biodot?

_____

_____

_____

4. What are some other measurements that could indicate increased stress that would be more reliable than the Biodot?

_____

_____

_____

5. What type of relaxation technique could you use during stressful activities?

_____

_____

_____

Understanding Clinical Trials

Using the following Internet link, read about clinical trials in NCCIH being conducted by the National Institutes of Health. Then, answer the following questions.

http://nccih.nih.gov/research/clinicaltrials/

1. What is a clinical trial?

_____

_____

_____

2. What are the common elements of a clinical trial?

_____

_____

_____

3. What is a placebo?

_____

_____

_____

277

4. What are the benefits and risks of participating in a clinical trial?

_____

_____

_____

Research a Clinical Trial

Using the following Internet link, investigate a NCCIH clinical trial being conducted by the National Institutes of Health. Write a paragraph describing the clinical trial. Include the purpose (intended outcome), supporting data, and your evaluation of the method being studied. Then, provide the missing information in the table.
https://www.nccih.nih.gov/research/clinicaltrials

_____

_____

_____

_____

_____

_____

_____

_____

_____

_____

_____

_____

_____

Clinical Trial

Description of the study	
Eligibility criteria for participants	
Length of the study	
Location of organization or parties completing the study	
Domain of CIH	

CRITICAL THINKING

1. List the advantages and disadvantages of one complementary or alternative health occupation including the following factors: job opportunities, salary range, fringe benefits, working conditions, occupational hazards, and educational requirements.
2. A group of practitioners in the United States call themselves certified naturopaths. They have not completed the training and education of the licensed naturopathic physician. Explain how a consumer can be confident about the training of a practitioner, and what could be done to remedy the confusion between these two branches of practitioners.

3. Create a career ladder for CAM careers. Describe why it is or is not possible to move from one level to another in the field.

4. You ask a patient which medications he is taking. He says only aspirin for an occasional headache. He asks if you want to know about his supplements, such as St. John's wort. What should you say?

5. Your friend tells you that she does not believe that any complementary or alternative therapies are useful. What should you say?

6. Your patient tells you that she has been using only complementary and alternative medicine (CAM) for her baby since birth. What should you say?

7. Your friend tells you he read an herbal cancer treatment on the Internet and wants your opinion about it. What should you say?

34 Forensic and Mortuary Science Professionals

CAREERS

Careers, Duties, and Credentials

Using the chapter and other sources, fill in the missing information.

CAREER TITLE	EDUCATION	DESCRIPTION OF JOB DUTIES	LICENSURE	CREDENTIALS
Pathologists' assistant			Certification via one of 11 accredited programs; exam	
		Helps with the physical movement of bodies to the funeral home; handles clerical duties; runs errands; arranges physical details of memorial service; may manage service		None
	Associate degree	Responsible for physical movement of decedent from place of death to final disposition; works with family and friends of the decedent to coordinate memorial services and provide support; submit required paperwork for death certificate; coordinate death benefits		
Embalmer			State licensure (except in CO)	
		Assists law enforcement agencies by processing evidence found during the investigation of a crime scene and writes reports of those findings		

Education Costs and Earnings Potential

Using the Internet, research the educational cost of one forensic and mortuary science career and the salary that might be earned in the local area. Use the information to complete the table.

CAREER	INSTITUTION FOR EDUCATION	COST OF EDUCATION	POTENTIAL EARNINGS

Skills and Qualities

Choose a career discussed in the chapter. List three personal qualities and skills that you think are important for the job and the reason(s) why.

1. _____

2. _____

3. _____

Exploring Career Opportunities

Many professional associations list career opportunities on their websites. Using one of the professional association links at the end of Chapter 34 in the textbook, search for job openings and locate the information requested below.

1. What professional association website did you choose?

   _____

2. How did you find job openings on that site?

   _____

   _____

3. Choose a posted job opening to explore. What is the job title? Where is it located?

   _____

   _____

   _____

4. What are the requirements for the job? What is the compensation and/or other benefits, if listed?

   _____

   _____

   _____

   _____

   _____

5. Discuss whether this job appeals to you. Why or why not?

   _____

   _____

   _____

   _____

   _____

Researching an Accredited Program

Using the Internet link http://www.abfse.org/, investigate a program accredited by the American Board of Funeral Service Education. You may be assigned a state in which to search, or you may select one on your own.

   Provide the name and address of the program, the degree(s) offered, and the following information for the most recent year available: number of enrollees, graduation rate, and the percentage of graduates employed in funeral science (FS). Also record the most recent 3-year averages for percentages of students passing the Arts and Science portions of the National Board Exam.

Name and address of program	
Degree(s) offered	
Number of enrollees	
Graduation rate	

Percentage of students employed in FS	
National Board Statistics: Average percentage of students who passed Arts	
National Board Statistics: Average percentage of students who passed Science	

Discuss whether this is a program you would be interested in attending. Why or why not?

_____

_____

_____

_____

_____

KNOWLEDGE CHECK

Multiple Choice

Circle the one correct answer to each of the following questions.

1. _____ care aims to make the terminally ill patient more comfortable, without attempting to cure the individual.
   a. Hospice
   b. Long-term
   c. Compassionate
   d. Geriatric

2. What is the course of study that prepares an individual to be a funeral service professional?
   a. Forensic pathology
   b. Burial science
   c. Mortuary science
   d. Histology

3. What is the term for the deceased person?
   a. Decedent
   b. Expiree
   c. Mortem
   d. Postmortem

4. What is the term for a body that has been donated for research?
   a. Decedent
   b. Shell
   c. Cadaver
   d. Specimen

5. Which of the following is a responsibility of a funeral director?
   a. Physical movement of the body
   b. Pronouncing time and manner of death
   c. Coordinating hospice care for the terminally ill
   d. Determining cause of death

6. Who declares a person legally dead?
   a. Physician
   b. Funeral director
   c. The first person to find the body
   d. Police

7. According to the Uniform Determination of Death Act (UDDA), one way death is determined is when there is an irreversible cessation of _____ function.
   a. kidney
   b. brain
   c. bowel
   d. immune

8. Which is another term for a funeral director?
   a. Coroner
   b. Pathologist
   c. Orderly
   d. Undertaker

9. What is the meaning of the term autopsy?
   a. Medical training
   b. A common burial method
   c. A technique to preserve the deceased
   d. A medical procedure to determine cause of death

10. Forensic pathology is the medical study of the body as it relates to
    a. legal processes.
    b. the surrounding environment.
    c. health.
    d. trauma.

11. Which career does not require a degree?
    a. Embalmer
    b. Funeral Attendant
    c. Pathologist's assistant
    d. Medical examiner

12. Dan studied biology in college, and then went on for two more years of school. In his master's program, he did clinical rotations and his coursework included medical photography. What is Dan's profession?
    a. Medical examiner
    b. Embalmer
    c. Funeral Attendant
    d. Pathologist's assistant

13. What is the meaning of the term *rigor mortis*?
    a. A condition associated with retaining fluid after death
    b. A common bacteria found in decedents
    c. A jelly-like condition of the organs and body tissue that occurs postmortem
    d. The stiffness that occurs in the body after death

14. Which technique is used to slow down the natural decomposition process?
    a. Cremation
    b. Embalming
    c. Postmortem examination
    d. Autopsy

15. The length of time an embalmed body can be stored depends on how well the body was embalmed as well as
    a. state law.
    b. the sex of the deceased.
    c. the manner or cause of death.
    d. ambient temperature and humidity.

16. What instrument is used to remove gasses and fluids from the abdominal cavity of the decedent?
    a. Forceps
    b. Scalpel
    c. Trocar
    d. Extractor

17. Regardless of the method of disposition, the first step in preparation is always
    a. using a trocar to inject embalming fluids.
    b. massaging the muscle tissue to relax rigor mortis.
    c. thoroughly washing the body.
    d. draining the blood from the body.

284

18. Cremation results in "ashes," which are predominantly
    a. starch.
    b. protein chains.
    c. desiccated cellular material.
    d. bone fragments.

19. What acts as a paper trail to ensure that remains or cremains are handled properly and according to the survivors wishes?
    a. Disposition permit
    b. Death certificate
    c. Patient medical records
    d. Living will

20. Which organization sets guidelines for funerary practices and enforces consumer protections?
    a. Centers for Disease Control and Prevention (CDC)
    b. Federal Trade Commission (FTC)
    c. American Medical Association (AMA)
    d. Office of the Attorney General (OAG)

True/False

Read the following statements and write "T" for true or "F" for false in the blanks provided. If a statement is false, correct the statement to make it true.

_____ 1. Vital records are the government's record of the events that happen in the lives of the population.
_____ 2. Mortuary science is the application of scientific techniques to criminal investigation.
_____ 3. In some counties, the coroner is elected, and in others it is an appointed position.
_____ 4. Most funeral homes have embalming and cremation areas on site.
_____ 5. As of 2021, funeral directors are licensed in all 50 states.
_____ 6. Regardless of job title, coroners and medical examiners have the same core job.
_____ 7. The coroner or medical examiner may order an autopsy.
_____ 8. The term *final disposition* refers to how the remains are to exist, such as burial or cremation.
_____ 9. State laws require every operating funeral home to have a designated preparation room.
_____ 10. The coroner or medical examiner completes and files the death certificate with the county or state.

CONTENT INSTRUCTION

Understanding the Concepts

Using your own words, answer each question in two or three sentences.

1. What guidelines for funeral homes does the Occupational Safety and Health Administration (OSHA) have, and why?

_____

_____

_____

_____

_____

_____

_____

2. What are some of the variables involved in the length of time it takes to cremate a human body?

_____

_____

_____

_____

_____

_____

3. What are some purposes that a donated body, or cadaver, might be used for by medical students?

_____

_____

_____

_____

PERFORMANCE INSTRUCTION

Reviewing a Death Certificate

Examine the portion of the example death certificate in Figure 34-1, then answer the following questions.

CAUSE OF DEATH (See instructions and examples)

		Approximate interval: Onset to death
32. PART I. Enter the chain of events--diseases, injuries, or complications--that directly caused the death. DO NOT enter terminal events such as cardiac arrest, respiratory arrest, or ventricular fibrillation without showing the etiology. DO NOT ABBREVIATE. Enter only one cause on a line. Add additional lines if necessary.		
IMMEDIATE CAUSE (Final disease or condition -------> resulting in death)	a. Aspiration pneumonia Due to (or as a consequence of):	2 Days
Sequentially list conditions, if any, leading to the cause listed on line a. Enter the UNDERLYING CAUSE (disease or injury that initiated the events resulting in death) LAST	b. Complications of coma Due to (or as a consequence of):	7 weeks
	c. Blunt force injuries Due to (or as a consequence of):	7 weeks
	d. Motor vehicle accident	7 weeks

PART II. Enter other significant conditions contributing to death but not resulting in the underlying cause given in PART I	33. WAS AN AUTOPSY PERFORMED? ■ Yes ☐ No
	34. WERE AUTOPSY FINDINGS AVAILABLE TO COMPLETE THE CAUSE OF DEATH? ■ Yes ☐ No

35. DID TOBACCO USE CONTRIBUTE TO DEATH? ☐ Yes ☐ Probably ■ No ☐ Unknown	36. IF FEMALE: ☐ Not pregnant within past year ☐ Pregnant at time of death ☐ Not pregnant, but pregnant within 42 days of death ☐ Not pregnant, but pregnant 43 days to 1 year before death ☐ Unknown if pregnant within the past year	37. MANNER OF DEATH ☐ Natural ☐ Homicide ■ Accident ☐ Pending Investigation ☐ Suicide ☐ Could not be determined

38. DATE OF INJURY (Mo/Day/Yr) (Spell Month) August 15, 2003	39. TIME OF INJURY Approx. 2320	40. PLACE OF INJURY (e.g., Decedent's home; construction site; restaurant; wooded area) road side near state highway	41. INJURY AT WORK? ☐ Yes ■ No

42. LOCATION OF INJURY: State: Missouri	City or Town: near Alexandria	
Street & Number: mile marker 17 on state route 46a	Apartment No.:	Zip Code:

43. DESCRIBE HOW INJURY OCCURRED: Decedent driver of van, ran off road into tree	44. IF TRANSPORTATION INJURY, SPECIFY: ■ Driver/Operator ☐ Passenger ☐ Pedestrian ☐ Other (Specify)

Figure 34-1 Death certificate.

1. What happened to the individual that caused the physician to declare the patient legally dead?

_____

_____

2. How long did the individual live after the car accident?

_____

3. Why do you think it is important to record the location of injury as opposed to the place of death?

_____

_____

_____

CRITICAL THINKING

1. Why is the accurate completion of the death certificate and disposition permit important?

_____

_____

_____

_____

_____

_____

_____

_____

_____

_____

2. Forensic science technicians have three distinct work environments: the laboratory, the legal setting, and the field. What are some examples of the type of work a forensic science technician does in each setting? Which environment do you think would be most challenging for you? Why?

_____

_____

_____

_____

_____

_____

_____

_____

_____

_____

287

35 Social and Mental Health Careers

Careers, Duties, and Credentials

Using the chapter and other sources, fill in the missing information.

CAREER TITLE	EDUCATION	DESCRIPTION OF JOB DUTIES	LICENSURE	CREDENTIALS
		Performs assessment; diagnoses condition, needs, and risks; plans, implements, and evaluates treatment (with input from supervisors)		
		Plan, organize, and direct medically approved recreation programs in hospitals and other settings	Varies by type	R-DMT, BC-DMT, MT-BC, others vary by state and type of therapy provided
	Medical school plus residency		State license	
	2 years postgraduate, minimum of 2 years supervised clinical experience	Evaluate patient and form diagnosis; provide psychotherapy	National exam, state licensure	
	Personal experience, training		Most states have a certification program; national certification once state certification obtained	

Education Costs and Earnings Potential

Using the Internet, research the educational cost of one social and mental health career and the salary that might be earned in the local area. Use the information to complete the table.

CAREER	INSTITUTION FOR EDUCATION	COST OF EDUCATION	POTENTIAL EARNINGS

Skills and Qualities

Choose a career discussed in the chapter. List three personal qualities and skills that you think are important for the job and the reason(s) why.

1. _____

2. _____

3. _____

289

Multiple Choice

Circle the correct answer to each question.

1. Which mental health professionals serve in a case management function?
   a. Psychiatrists
   b. Expressing therapists
   c. Psychiatric technicians
   d. Social workers

2. Prescriptive authority means
   a. a provider has the legal power to write prescriptions.
   b. a patient can take as many drugs as they need.
   c. a nurse can prescribe medications in an emergency.
   d. a patient believes he is in charge of the health care facility.

3. A registered nurse (RN) needs which certification to work in the psychiatric setting?
   a. NCLEX-RN
   b. PMH-APRN
   c. Psy.D.
   d. None

4. What is an expressive therapist?
   a. A mental health professional who leads group sessions and makes home visits
   b. A mental health professional who uses arts, movement and crafts to assist in the healing process
   c. A mental health professional who assists patients with activities of daily living
   d. A mental health professional who coordinates care and assesses needs such as housing

5. The field of science that studies the relationship of the function of the brain to psychological behavior is
   a. psychology.
   b. psychoanalysis.
   c. neurobiology.
   d. psychiatry.

6. The _____ identifies the exact symptoms necessary to make a mental diagnosis.
   a. ICD-9
   b. ICD-10
   c. CM-PCS
   d. DSM-5

7. What is the term for an individual turning to drugs and alcohol to relieve symptoms of his or her mental illness?
   a. Self-medicating
   b. Compulsion
   c. Impulsivity
   d. Obsessing

8. What disorder that sometimes features mood swings, headaches, and flashbacks can develop after witnessing or experiencing a terrifying, violent event?
   a. Antisocial personality disorder
   b. Post-traumatic stress disorder (PTSD)
   c. Obsessive-compulsive disorder (OCD)
   d. Major depressive disorder (MDD)

9. What is the term for persistent, unwanted thoughts, and images?
   a. Obsessions
   b. Compulsions
   c. Mania
   d. Depression

10. What is the term for hearing voices or seeing things that are not real?
    a. Disorganized thinking
    b. Delusion
    c. Hallucinations
    d. Mania

11. Patients in a mental health crisis usually stay in inpatient acute setting for _____.
    a. 5–7 days
    b. 12–36 hours
    c. 1–3 days
    d. 30 days
12. What is the term for isolating a person in a room that they cannot leave?
    a. Admission
    b. Confinement
    c. Seclusion
    d. Inpatient
13. Calendars, clocks, and a routine for daily activities can keep the patient
    a. oriented.
    b. confused.
    c. confined.
    d. isolated.
14. Which type of facility treats patients who cannot access private practice providers?
    a. Substance abuse treatment centers
    b. Community mental health centers
    c. Emergency departments (EDs) in hospitals
    d. Self-employed psychologist's offices
15. Which form of rehabilitation promotes awareness of person, place, and time?
    a. Reality orientation
    b. Isolation
    c. Restraint
    d. Electroconvulsive therapy (ECT)

True/False
Read the following statements and write "T" for true or "F" for false in the blanks provided. If a statement is false, correct the statement to make it true.

_____ 1. Employee assistance programs (EAPs) are a workplace benefit to help employees with personal and work-related challenges.

_____ 2. Registered dance therapists must complete graduate-level preparation and examination.

_____ 3. Some states do not require a license to function as a counselor in private practice and accept insurance.

_____ 4. Both psychiatrists and psychologist are considered medical doctors.

_____ 5. Mental illnesses can usually be diagnosed using a blood panel.

_____ 6. Some people with suicidal ideation, depending on their history, need not be taken too seriously.

_____ 7. Asperger's syndrome is classed on the autism spectrum, per the 5th edition of the DSM.

_____ 8. Many mental illnesses are treated in private practice.

_____ 9. Confusion may result from a reduced blood supply to the brain.

_____ 10. Electroconvulsive therapy (ECT) must be performed when patient is awake and alert.

CONTENT INSTRUCTION

Defining the Concepts
Using your own words, define each term or concept in one to three sentences.

1. Neuroplasticity

_____

_____

_____

2. Substance use disorder

_____

_____

_____

3. Body dysmorphic disorder

_____

_____

_____

4. Bulimia nervosa

_____

_____

_____

5. Psychosis

_____

_____

_____

PERFORMANCE APPLICATIONS

Using Progressive Muscle Relaxation

Choose a partner. Each of you will take a turn being the director and the participant. Read all the instructions before beginning this activity. Laboratory activities should be completed under the supervision of a qualified professional only.

Equipment and Supplies

Comfortable area, ideally with dimmable lights

Directions

1. Instruct your classmate to recline, relax, and to remain still so as not to engage any muscles.
2. Direct your classmate to focus on the muscles of the arms and hands.
3. Instruct your classmate to tense the muscle group for 5 seconds, breathe in and out, then quickly relax.
4. Have your classmate reflect on the sensations of relaxation for 10–20 seconds.
5. Repeat the process for the face and neck.
6. Repeat the process for the chest, shoulders, back, and abdomen.
7. Repeat the process for the legs and feet.
8. Record the information in the table as indicated.

TIME OF READING	SELF-IDENTIFIED LEVEL OF STRESS ON SCALE OF 1–5 (1 = no stress, 5 = highest stress)
Before exercise	
After exercise	

Questions

1. How did you determine who would direct the initial progressive muscle relaxation exercise (director) and who would follow the directions (participant)?

_____

_____

_____

2. Did you feel more stressed as the director or as the participant?

_____

_____

_____

3. Did you perceive a lessened stress level when you engaged in progressive muscle relaxation as the participant?

_____

_____

_____

4. What are some factors that you think might make progressive muscle relaxation effective?

_____

_____

_____

5. What mental disorders may be helped with the use of progressive muscle relaxation?

_____

_____

_____

Locating Mental Health Services

Using the following Internet link, locate mental health services available near you. Then, answer the following questions.
https://www.samhsa.gov

1. What type of mental health services did you look for?

_____

_____

2. How did you use the website to locate mental health services near you?

_____

_____

_____

3. What treatment types were discussed?

_____

_____

_____

_____

293

4. Choose one facility. What services are offered, and what payment is accepted for them?

_____

_____

_____

_____

_____

_____

_____

Research a Clinical Trial

Using the following Internet link, investigate a National Institute of Mental Health clinical trial. Write a paragraph describing the clinical trial process. Include the purpose (intended outcome), supporting data, and your evaluation of the method being studied. Then provide the missing information in the table.
https://www.mentalhealth.gov/get-help/clinical-trial

_____

_____

_____

_____

_____

_____

_____

_____

_____

_____

_____

_____

_____

_____

Clinical Trial

Description of the study	
Eligibility criteria for participants	
Length of the study	
Location of organization or parties completing the study	

Research Medical Treatments

Investigate five common medications used in mental health care treatments. Discuss the indications, contraindications, and side effects of each.

_____

_____

_____

_____

_____

_____

_____

_____

_____

_____

_____

_____

_____

CRITICAL THINKING

1. Use the Internet to research the risk and protective factors associated with suicide. Compare and contrast the following terms: suicidal ideation, suicide attempt, and suicide.

_____

_____

_____

_____

_____

_____

_____

_____

_____

_____

295

2. You are assigned to a patient who is confused and thinks you are her daughter. What should you do?

_____

_____

_____

_____

3. Your patient tells you he is going to quit taking his medication for depression because it makes him feel confused. What should you say?

_____

_____

_____

_____

4. Your friend has been giving her things away, saying goodbye to you and others, and talking about suicide. What should you do?

_____

_____

_____

_____

5. You observe that your friend has many relationships that do not last very long. When you talk about it, she says that she feels that all the men she meets want to control her. She says she hates herself for that feeling. What should you say?

_____

_____

_____

_____